EVIDENCE-BASED
MEDICINE

How to Practice and Teach EBM

DEDICATIONS

This book is dedicated to Dr David L. Sackett
and to the memory of Dr Hui Lee

Commissioning Editor: Michael Parkinson
Project Development Manager: Janice Urquhart
Project Manager: Frances Affleck
Designer: Judith Wright
Illustration Manager: Bruce Hogarth
Illustrator: Robert Britton

EVIDENCE-BASED
MEDICINE

How to Practice and Teach EBM

Sharon E. Straus
Associate Professor, University Health Network,
University of Toronto, Toronto, Ontario, Canada

W. Scott Richardson
Director, Three Owl Learning Institute and Associate Professor of
Medicine, Wright State University School of Medicine, Dayton, Ohio, USA

Paul Glasziou
Director, Centre for Evidence-Based Practice, University of Oxford,
Oxford, UK

R. Brian Haynes
Professor of Clinical Epidemiology and Medicine, McMaster University,
Hamilton, Ontario, Canada

THIRD EDITION

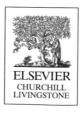

ELSEVIER
CHURCHILL
LIVINGSTONE

EDINBURGH LONDON NEW YORK OXFORD PHILADELPHIA ST LOUIS SYDNEY TORONTO
2005

ELSEVIER
CHURCHILL
LIVINGSTONE

First edition 1997
Second edition 2000
Third edition 2005

ISBN 0 443 07444 5

British Library Cataloguing in Publication Data
A catalogue record for this book is available from the British Library

Library of Congress Cataloging in Publication Data
A catalog record for this book is available from the Library of Congress

Note
Medical knowledge is constantly changing. Standard safety precautions
must be followed, but as new research and clinical experience broaden our
knowledge, changes in treatment and drug therapy may become necessary
or appropriate. Readers are advised to check the most current product
information provided by the manufacturer of each drug to be
administered to verify the recommended dose, the method and duration
of administration, and contraindications. It is the responsibility of the
practitioner, relying on experience and knowledge of the patient,
to determine dosages and the best treatment for each individual patient.
Neither the Publisher nor the authors assume any liability for any injury
and/or damage to persons or property arising from this publication.

The Publisher

 **your source for books,
journals and multimedia
in the health sciences**

www.elsevierhealth.com

The
publisher's
policy is to use
paper manufactured
from sustainable forests

Printed in China

Resources that accompany this text

The accompanying compact disk

The chapters and appendices that comprise this book constitute a traditional way of presenting our ideas about EBM. We wanted to keep this book pocket-sized and therefore our discussion is restricted by the limits of print space. To overcome this limitation, we've provided additional materials on the accompanying CD, including resources for practicing EBM that can be downloaded to your PDA. The CD also contains clinical examples, critical appraisals, and background papers from other health care disciplines, including nursing and occupational therapy, and links to various evidence resources.

Minimum system requirements

Windows®

Windows 98 or higher
Pentium® processor-based PC
16 MB RAM (32 MB recommended)
10 MB of available hard-disk space
2 X or faster CD-ROM drive
VGA monitor supporting thousands of colours (16-bit)

Macintosh®

Apple Power Macintosh
Mac OS version 9 or later
64 MB of available RAM
10 MB of available hard-disk space
2 X or faster CD-ROM drive
NB: NO data are transferred to the hard disk.
The CD-ROM is self-contained and the application runs directly from the CD-ROM.

Installation instructions

Macintosh

If you have enabled CD-ROM autoplay on your system then the CD-ROM will run automatically when inserted into your CD-ROM drive. If you have not enabled autoplay, click on the CD-ROM icon that appears on your desktop, then click on 'Straus' to open the application.

To enable the CD-ROM to autorun, select the Control Panels from the Apple menu on your desktop. Select QuickTime settings, then select Autoplay. Click the Enable CD-ROM Autoplay checkbox, and then save the settings.

Windows
If you have enabled CD-ROM autoplay on your system then the CD-ROM will run automatically when inserted into your CD-ROM drive. If you have not enabled autoplay, click on My Computer and double-click on your CD-Rom drive. Your CD-ROM drive should be represented by an icon labeled 'Straus'.

Using this product
This product is designed to run with Internet Explorer 5.0 or later (PC) and Netscape 4.5 or later (Mac). Please refer to the help files on those programs for problems specific to the browser.

Viewing images
1. **Viewing the images by chapter**
   From the table of contents, click on an individual chapter to view images. Corresponding legends are provided alongside each image. By clicking on the image an enlarged image can be viewed in a new window. The image can also be viewed in PDF format using the link 'view PDF'.

2. **Selecting the images for presentation**
   Click on the link 'Add to presentation' provided below each image to add it to the presentation. As soon as you add an image to your presentation, a window will pop up showing the list of all selected images as slides. In that window you can preview all the slides selected for presentation using the links Slide#. To remove a slide from the presentation click on the ❑ image.

3. Export

a) PowerPoint Presentation:
The selected images can be exported and saved as a Microsoft PowerPoint presentation. This feature is available in Microsoft Windows Operating Systems having full version of Microsoft PowerPoint only.

b) HTML Presentation:
The selected images can be saved as an HTML presentation for users without Microsoft PowerPoint. This feature is available in both Microsoft Windows and Macintosh Operating Systems.

On MacOS, the HTML Presentation is saved directly in the Hard drive

Note: For more details, please refer to the 'Help' section on the CD-Rom.

To use some of the functions on the CD, the user must have the following:

1. CD requires "Java Runtime Environment" to be installed in your system to use "Export" and "Slide Show" features. CD automatically checks for "Java Runtime Environment" version 1.3.1 or later (PC) and MRJ 2.2.5 (Mac) if not available, it starts installing from the CD. Please complete the installation process. Then click on the license agreement to proceed. "Java Runtime Environment" is available in the CD's Software folder. If the user manually installs the software, please make sure that the user starts the application by clicking 'Straus.exe'.

2. Your browser needs to be Java-enabled. If the user did not enable Java when installing your browser, the user may need to download some additional files from your browser manufacturer.

3. If your system does not support Autorun, then please explore the CD contents, click on 'Straus.exe' to start.

Acrobat Reader can be installed from the Software folder of the CD.

Technical support

Technical support for this product is available between 7:30 a.m. and 7 p.m. CST, Monday through Friday. Before calling, be sure that your computer meets the minimum system requirements to run this software. Inside the United States and Canada, call 1-800-692-9010. Inside the United Kingdom, call 0080069290100. Outside North America, call +1-314-872-8370. You may also fax your questions to +1-314-997-5080, or contact Technical Support through e-mail: *technical.support@elsevier.com.*

The book's website

http://www.cebm.utoronto.ca
Because the examples used in this book will be out of date by the time you're reading this, the supporting website for this book (given above) will provide updates and new materials, so we'd suggest you check it periodically. It will also be a means of contacting the authors and letting us know where we've gone wrong and what we could do better in the future.

Icons

This icon highlights teaching methods described in the text.

This icon indicates that there is a link between the text and the coloured cards to be found in the cover pocket.

Contents

The CD

CONTENTS

A Evidence-based medicine: how to practice and teach EBM

B Practicing and teaching evidence-based health care in other clinical specialities

1. General internal medicine
- Introduction to evidence-based internal medicine
- Other resources for evidence-based internal medicine
- Sample scenarios, searches and completed worksheets:
  - ➤ Diagnosis (iron deficiency anemia)
  - ➤ Therapy (statins)
  - ➤ Prognosis (mitral valve prolapse)
  - ➤ Harm (caffeine and urinary incontinence)
  - ➤ Systematic reviews (donepezil and Alzheimer's dementia)

2. Evidence-based nursing
- Introduction to evidence-based nursing
- Other resources for evidence-based nursing
- Sample scenarios, search strategies, completed worksheets and CATs for evidence-based nursing

- ➢ Diagnosis (depression)
- ➢ Prognosis (grief after pregnancy loss)
- ➢ Therapy (zinc lozenges)
- ➢ Harm (oral contraceptives)
- ➢ Systematic reviews (asthma and self-management education)
- ➢ Qualitative research (long-term care studies)

3. *Occupational therapy*
   - Introduction to evidence-based occupational therapy
   - Other resources for evidence-based occupational therapy
   - Sample scenarios, searches and critical appraisal worksheets

4. *Appendix: Critical appraisal worksheets*

C Evidence resources
   - Criteria for inclusion of evidence resources
   - Journals
   - Textbooks
   - CDs
   - Websites

D EBM toolbox
   - GATE critical appraisal worksheets
   - Educational prescription
   - Search cascade
   - CATMaker
   - Pocket cards
   - Annotated bibliography

E PDA tools
   - EBM calculator
   - NNT/LR tables
   - Pocket cards
   - Educational prescription
   - CQ log

Preface

This book is for clinicians at any stage of their training or career who want to learn how to practice and teach evidence-based medicine (EBM). It's been written for the busy clinician, thus it's short and practical. This book emphasizes direct clinical application of EBM and tactics to practice EBM in real-time. Those who wish, and have time for, more detailed discussions of the theoretical and methodological bases for the tactics described here should consult one of the longer textbooks on clinical epidemiology.*

The focus of the book has changed with the continuing clinical experiences of the authors. For Sharon Straus, the ideas behind the ongoing development of the book have built on her experiences as a medical student on a general medicine ward, when she was challenged by a senior resident to provide evidence to support her management plans for each patient she admitted. This was so much more exciting than some previous rotations, where the management plan was learned by rote and was based on whatever the current consultant favored. After residency, she undertook postgraduate training in clinical epidemiology and this further stimulated her interest in EBM, leading to a fellowship with Dave Sackett in Oxford. While there her enthusiasm for practicing and teaching EBM continued to grow. She hopes that this has led to improved patient care and to more fun and challenge for her students and residents, from whom she's learned so much.

For Paul Glasziou, the first inkling of another way began when, as a newly qualified and puzzled doctor, he was fortunate enough to stumble on a copy of Henrik Wulff's *Rational Diagnosis*

---

* The ones we consult are the third edition of *Clinical Epidemiology, The Essentials* (Fletcher R H, Fletcher S W, Wagner E H. Baltimore: Williams & Wilkins, 1996), *Clinical Epidemiology and Biostatistics* (Kramer M S. Berlin: Springer-Verlag, 1988), and the second edition of *Clinical Epidemiology: A Basic Science for Clinical Medicine* (Sackett D L, Haynes R B, Guyatt G H, Tugwell P. Boston: Little Brown, 1991). Note that this latter book is currently being rewritten and we'd suggest you visit *www.davesackett.com* to find out further details.

and Treatment. After a long journey of exploration (thanks Arthur, Jorgen, John, and Les), a serendipitous visit from Dave Sackett to Sydney in the late 1980s led him to return to clinical work. An all too brief visit to McMaster University with Dave Sackett convinced him that research *really* could be used to improve care on the ward. Feeling better armed to recognize and manage the uncertainties inherent in medical consultations, he continues to enjoy general practice, and teaching others to record and answer their own clinical questions. He remains awed by the vast unexplored tracts of clinical practice not visible from the eyepiece of a microscope. Rather than write "what I never learnt at medical school" he is delighted to contribute to this book.

For Scott Richardson, the ideas for this book began coming together very slowly. As a clinical clerk in the 1970s, one of his teachers told him to read an article to decide what to do for his patient, but then said "Of course, nobody really does that!" During residency, Scott tried harder to use the literature but found few tools to help him do it effectively. Some of the ideas for this book took shape for Scott when he came across the notions of clinical epidemiology and critical appraisal in the late 1970s and early 1980s and he began to use them in his practice and teaching of students and postgraduates at the University of Rochester. On his journey in Rochester, Hamilton, Oxford, San Antonio, Dayton, and elsewhere, Scott has worked with others in EBM (including these co-authors), fashioning those earlier ideas into clinician-friendly tools for everyday use. Scott continues to have heap big fun learning from and teaching with a large number of EBM colleagues around the world, all working to improve the care of patients by making wise use of research evidence.

Brian Haynes started worrying about the relationship between evidence and clinical practice during his second year of medical school when a psychiatrist gave a lecture on Freud's theories. When asked, "What's the evidence that Freud's theories were correct?", the psychiatrist admitted that there wasn't any good evidence, and that he didn't believe the theories, but he had been asked by the head of the department "to give the talk". This eventually led Brian to a career combining clinical practice with research in clinical epidemiology to "get the evidence", only to find that the evidence being generated by medical researchers around the world wasn't getting to practitioners and patients in a timely and dependable way. Sabbaticals permitted a career shift into medical informatics to look into how knowledge is disseminated and applied, and how practitioners and patients can use and benefit from "current best evidence". This led to the development of several evidence-based information resources, including ACP Journal Club, Evidence-Based Medicine, Evidence-Based Nursing, Evidence-Based Mental Health, in print and electronic versions, to make it easier for practitioners to get at the best current evidence. At present, he is devising even more devious ways to get evidence into practice, including making highly refined evidence so inexpensive and available that less-refined evidence won't stand a chance in competing for practitioners' reading materials, computers or brains. They also say that he's a dreamer...

A note about our choice of words: we'll talk about "our" patients throughout this book, not to imply any possession or control of them by us, but to signify that we have taken on an obligation and responsibility to care for and serve each of them. We're sure that this book contains several errors – we just don't know (yet!) what and where they are. When you find them, please jump on our website and tell us about them. In return, we'll credit your eagle eyes on the website and in subsequent printings of the book.

For the contents of this book to benefit patients, we believe that clinicians must have a mastery of the clinical skills, including history-taking, and physical examination, without which we can neither begin the process of EBM (by generating diagnostic hypotheses) nor end it (by integrating valid, important evidence with our patients' values and expectations). We also advocate continuous, self-directed lifelong learning. As T. H. White wrote in *The Once and Future King*, "Learning is the only thing which the mind can never exhaust, never alienate, never be tortured by, never fear or distrust, and never dream of regretting". By not regarding knowledge with humility and by denying our uncertainty and curiosity, we risk becoming dangerously out of date and immune to self-improvement and advances in medicine. Finally, we implore you to add the enthusiasm and irreverence to the endeavor without which you will miss the fun that accompanies the application of these ideas!

Acknowledgements

If this book is found to be useful, much of the credit for it is due to Muir Gray and David L. Sackett who created and led, respectively, the NHS R&D Centre for Evidence-Based Practice at Oxford, which has provided a home and working retreat for all of the authors at various times. They have provided the authors with great mentorship, and advice including, "If you can dream it, you can do it". And so, we thank them for encouraging us to dream, and for helping us to achieve those dreams.

We thank our colleagues for their infinite patience and our families for their loving support. Sharon Straus gives special thanks to Eliot Phillipson and Maria Bacchus for their support, to all her students, fellows and residents for their inspiration and fun, and to Dave Sackett for his friendship and mentoring. Paul Glasziou would like to thank Arthur Elstein, Jorgen Hilden, John Simes, Les Irwig, and Dave Sackett for their mentorship and friendship. Scott Richardson gives special thanks to Sherry Parmer and her daughter Alexandra, and to his many teachers and colleagues who have taught by example and who have given him so generously both intellectual challenge and personal support. Brian Haynes thanks the American College of Physicians and the BMJ Publishing Group for leading the way in providing opportunities to create and disseminate many of the "evidence-based" information resources featured in this book and its companion CD and website.

The number of individuals who gave wonderfully warm and candid feedback on the previous editions of the book now number in the thousands; we give special thanks to Yasuhiro Asai, Inke Konig, Eleftherios Anevlarius, Leon Collins, Tim Pauley, Barbara Roach, Anand Dale, Angie Fearon, Romuald Riem, Alan Adelman, Manon Bruinsma, Takahiro Okamoto, Hiroshi Noto, Raymond Leung, Evan Fung, and Jan Kejah. Colleagues who offered important suggestions for this edition include Michael Green, Eduardo Ortiz, Darlyne Rath, Jayne Holroyd-Leduc, and Rod Jackson.

We're still seeking better ways of explaining these ideas and their clinical application, and will acknowledge readers' suggestions in subsequent editions of this book. In the meantime, we take cheerful responsibility for the parts of the current edition that are still fuzzy, wrong, or boring.

WHAT IS EBM?

Evidence-based medicine (EBM) requires the integration of the best research evidence with our clinical expertise and our patient's unique values and circumstances.

- By *best research evidence* we mean valid and clinically relevant research, often from the basic sciences of medicine, but especially from patient-centered clinical research into the accuracy of diagnostic tests (including the clinical examination), the power of prognostic markers, and the efficacy and safety of therapeutic, rehabilitative, and preventive regimens. New evidence from clinical research both invalidates previously accepted diagnostic tests and treatments and replaces them with new ones that are more accurate, more efficacious, and safer.

- By *clinical expertise* we mean the ability to use our clinical skills and past experience to rapidly identify each patient's unique health state and diagnosis, their individual risks and benefits of potential interventions, and their personal circumstances and expectations.

- By *patient values* we mean the unique preferences, concerns and expectations each patient brings to a clinical encounter and which must be integrated into clinical decisions if they are to serve the patient.

- By *patient circumstances* we mean their individual clinical state and the clinical setting.

WHY THE INTEREST IN EBM?

Interest in EBM has grown exponentially since the coining of the term[1] in 1992 by a group led by Gordon Guyatt at McMaster University, from one MEDLINE citation in 1992 to over 13 000 in February 2004. Professional organizations and training programs for health care professionals have moved from whether to teach EBM to how to teach it, resulting in an explosion in the number of courses, workshops and seminars offered in this practice. Reports describing evidence-based rejuvenations of traditional educational events are burgeoning, and case reports and a survey of residency programs have concluded that some of the determinants of continuing high attendance at postgraduate journal clubs include the teaching of critical appraisal skills and emphasizing the primary literature (and, not surprisingly, providing free food).[2,3] Also, familiarity with EBM terminology has extended into the popular press, as evidenced by an article in *The Times* describing the number needed to treat.[4]

The rapid spread of EBM has arisen from four realizations and is made possible by five recent developments. The realizations, attested to by ever-increasing numbers of clinicians, are:

1. Our daily need for valid information about diagnosis, prognosis, therapy, and prevention (up to five times per inpatient[5] and twice for every three outpatients).[6]

2. The inadequacy of traditional sources for this information because they are out of date (textbooks[7]), frequently wrong (experts[8]), ineffective (didactic continuing medical education[9]), or too overwhelming in their volume and too variable in their validity for practical clinical use (medical journals[10]).

3. The disparity between our diagnostic skills and clinical judgment, which increase with experience, and our up-to-date knowledge[11] and clinical performance,[12] which decline.

4. Our inability to afford more than a few seconds per patient for finding and assimilating this evidence[13] or to set aside more than half an hour per week for general reading and study.[14]

Until recently, these problems were insurmountable for full-time clinicians. However, five developments have permitted a turnaround in this state of affairs:

1. The development of strategies for efficiently tracking down and appraising evidence (for its validity and relevance).

2. The creation of systematic reviews of the effects of health care (epitomized by the Cochrane Collaboration[15]).

3. The creation of evidence-based journals of secondary publication (which publish the 2% of clinical articles that are both valid and of immediate clinical use) and of evidence-based summary services such as Clinical Evidence.

4. The creation of information systems for bringing the foregoing to us in seconds.[13]

5. The identification and application of effective strategies for lifelong learning and for improving our clinical performance.[16]

This book is devoted to describing these innovations, demonstrating their application to clinical problems, and showing how they can be learned and practiced by clinicians who have just 30 minutes per week to devote to their continuing professional development.

HOW DO WE ACTUALLY PRACTICE EBM?

The full-blown practice of EBM comprises five steps; this book takes them up in turn:

- *Step 1*: converting the need for information (about prevention, diagnosis, prognosis, therapy, causation, etc.) into an answerable question (Ch. 1).

- *Step 2*: tracking down the best evidence with which to answer that question (Ch. 2).

- *Step 3*: critically appraising that evidence for its validity (closeness to the truth), impact (size of the effect), and applicability (usefulness in our clinical practice) (the first halves of Chs 3–6).

- *Step 4*: integrating the critical appraisal with our clinical expertise and with our patient's unique biology, values, and circumstances (the second halves of Chs 3–6).

- *Step 5*: evaluating our effectiveness and efficiency in executing steps 1–4 and seeking ways to improve them both for next time (Ch. 8).

When we examine our practice and that of our colleagues and trainees in this five-step fashion, we identify that clinicians can incorporate evidence into their practices in three ways. First, is the "doing" mode, in which at least the first four steps above are carried out. Second, is the "using" mode, in which searches are restricted to evidence resources that have already undergone critical appraisal by others, such as evidence summaries (thus skipping step 3). Third, is the "replicating" mode, in which the decisions of respected opinion leaders are followed (abandoning at least steps 2 and 3). All three of these modes involve the integration of evidence (from whatever source) with our patient's unique biology, values and circumstances of step 4, but they vary in the execution of the other steps.

For conditions we encounter every day (e.g. unstable angina and venous thromboembolism), we need to be "up-to-the-minute" and very sure about what we are doing. Accordingly, we invest the time and effort necessary to carry out both steps 2 (searching) and 3 (critically appraising), and operate in the "doing" mode; all the chapters in this book are relevant to this mode.

For conditions we encounter less often (e.g. aspirin overdose), we conserve our time by seeking out critical appraisals already performed by others who describe (and stick to!) explicit criteria for deciding what evidence they selected and how they decided whether it was valid. We leave out the time-consuming step 3 (critically appraising) and carry out just step 2 (searching) but restrict the latter to sources that have already undergone rigorous critical appraisal (e.g. *ACP Journal Club*). Only the third portions ("Can I apply this valid, important evidence to my patient?") of Chapters 3–6 are strictly relevant here, and the growing database of pre-appraised resources (described in Ch. 2 and on the accompanying CD) is making this "using" mode increasingly feasible for busy clinicians.

For the problems we're likely to encounter very infrequently (e.g. graft vs. host disease in a bone marrow transplant recipient), we "blindly" seek, accept, and apply the recommendations we receive from authorities in the relevant branch of medicine. This "replicating" mode also characterizes the practice of medical students and clinical trainees when they haven't yet been granted independence and have to carry out the orders of their consultants. The trouble with the "replicating" mode is that it is "blind" to whether the advice received from the experts is authoritative (evidence-based, resulting from their operating in the "appraising" mode) or merely authoritarian (opinion-based). Sometimes we can gain clues about the validity of our expert source (Do they cite references? Are they a member of the Cochrane Collaboration?), although this may require some probing ("Can you tell me the basis for that? Do you have a reference?"). If we tracked the care we give when operating in the "replicating" mode into the literature and critically appraised it, we would find that some of it was effective, some useless, and some harmful. But in the "replicating" mode we'll never be sure which.

The authors of this book don't practice as EBM doers all of the time and we find that we move between the different modes of practicing EBM depending on the clinical scenario, the frequency with which it arises, and the time and resources available to address our clinical questions. And, while some clinicians may want to become proficient in practicing all five steps of EBM, many others would instead prefer to focus on becoming efficient users (and knowledge managers) of evidence. This book tries to meet the needs of these various end-users. And, for those readers who are teachers of EBM, we try to describe various ways in which the learning needs of the different learners can be achieved, including those who want to be primarily users or doers of EBM.

CAN CLINICIANS ACTUALLY PRACTICE EBM?

Surveys conducted amongst clinicians from various disciplines have found that clinicians are interested in learning the necessary skills for practicing EBM.[17,18] One survey of UK GPs suggests that many clinicians already practice in the "using" mode, using evidence-based summaries generated by others (72%) and evidence-based practice guidelines or protocols (84%).[18] On the other hand, far fewer claimed to understand (and to be able to explain) the "appraising" tools of number needed to treat (NNT) (35%) and confidence intervals (20%). Interestingly, a recent study found that participants' self-ratings of their understanding of terms used in EBM (e.g. relative risk and NNT) differed substantially from an objective, criterion-based assessment.[19] Moreover, comments from participants reflected considerable misunderstanding of these terms.

If clinicians have the necessary skills for practicing EBM, can it be done in real-time? When a busy (180+ admissions per month) inpatient medical service brought electronic summaries of evidence previously appraised either by team members (critically appraised topics—CATs) or by summary journals to working rounds, it was documented that, on average, the former could be accessed in 10 seconds and the latter in 25.[13] Moreover, when assessed from the viewpoint of the most junior member of the team caring for the patient, this evidence changed 25% of their diagnostic and treatment suggestions and added to a further 23% of them. This study has been replicated in other clinical settings, including an obstetrical service.[20] Finally, clinical audits from several practice settings have found that there is a significant evidence base for the primary interventions that are encountered on these clinical services.[21–25]

WHAT'S THE "E" FOR EBM?

There is an accumulating body of evidence relating to the impact of EBM on health care professionals, from systematic reviews of training in the skills of EBM[26] to qualitative research describing the experience of EBM practitioners.[27] However, studies of the effect of teaching and practicing EBM are challenging to conduct. In many studies, the intervention has been difficult to define. It's unclear what the appropriate "dose", "formulation", "frequency" or "route" should be. Some studies use an approach to clinical practice, whereas others use training in one of the discrete "microskills" of EBM, such as MEDLINE searching[28] or critical appraisal. Moreover, learners have different learning needs and styles, and these differences must be reflected in the educational experiences provided.

Just as the intervention has proved difficult to define, the evaluation of whether the intervention has met its goals has been challenging. Effective EBM interventions will produce a wide range of outcomes. Changes in knowledge and skills are relatively easy to detect and demonstrate. Changes in attitudes and behaviors are harder to confirm. A recent study has shown that a multifaceted EBM educational intervention (including access to evidence resources and a seminar series using real clinical scenarios) significantly improved evidence-based practice patterns in a district general hospital.[29] Still more challenging is detecting changes in clinical outcomes. To date, studies demonstrating better patient survival when practice is evidence-based (and worse when it isn't) are limited to outcomes research.[30,31] No such evidence is available from randomized trials because no investigative team or research granting agency has yet overcome the problems of sample size, contamination, blinding, and long-term follow-up which such a trial requires. Moreover, there are ethical concerns with such a trial: is withholding access to evidence from the control clinicians ethical?

But, by questioning the "E" for EBM, are we asking the right question? It has been recognized that providing evidence from clinical research is a necessary but not sufficient condition for the provision of optimal care. This has created interest in knowledge translation, the scientific study of the methods for closing the knowledge-to-practice gap and the analysis of barriers and facilitators inherent in this process.[32] The process from knowledge to practice involves several stages, such as initial awareness, appraisal and acceptance, skill and ability in the new technique, reminder systems, and skilled communication with patients (Figure I.1). Proponents of knowledge translation have identified that changing behavior is a complex process requiring comprehensive approaches directed towards patients, physicians, managers, and policy-makers, and provision of evidence is but one component.[33] Finally, it may be too soon to tell if EBM changes clinical performance and outcomes, because advocates suggest that it requires lifelong learning and this is not something that can be measured over the short-term.

WHAT ARE THE LIMITATIONS OF EBM?

Discussion about the practice of EBM naturally engenders negative and positive reactions from clinicians. Some of the criticisms focus on misunderstandings and misperceptions of EBM, such as the concerns that it ignores patient values and preferences and promotes a cookbook approach.[34] An examination of the definition and steps of EBM quickly dismisses these criticisms. Others have expressed worry that EBM will be hijacked by managers to promote cost-cutting. However, EBM is not an effective cost-cutting tool, since providing evidence-based care directed toward maximizing patients' quality of life often increases the costs of their care and raises the ire of health economists.[35] The self-reported employment of the "using" mode by a great majority of front-line GPs dispels the contention that EBM is an ivory tower concept—another common criticism. Finally, we hope that the rest of this book will put to rest the concern that EBM leads to therapeutic nihilism in the absence of randomized trial evidence.

However, this debate has highlighted limitations unique to the practice of EBM that must be considered. For example,

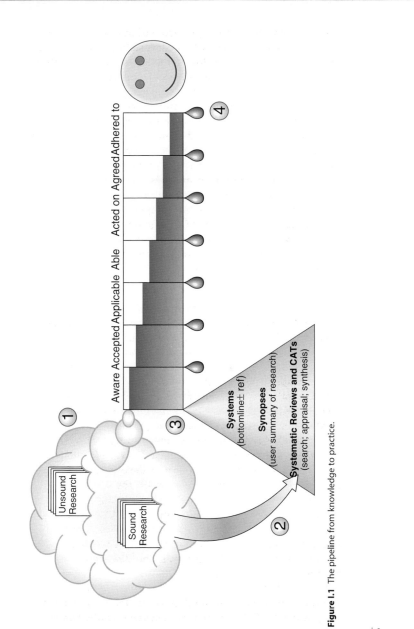

Figure I.1 The pipeline from knowledge to practice.

Aware Accepted Applicable Able Acted on Agreed Adhered to

① ②

Systems (bottomline± ref)
Synopses (user summary of research)
Systematic Reviews and CATs (search; appraisal; synthesis)

Unsound Research

Sound Research

③ ④

the need to develop new skills in seeking and appraising evidence cannot be underestimated. And the need to develop and apply these skills within the time constraints of our clinical practice must be addressed.

This book attempts to tackle these limitations and offers potential solutions. For example, EBM skills can be acquired at any stage in clinical training, and members of clinical teams at various stages of training can collaborate by sharing the searching and appraising tasks. Incorporating the acquisition of these skills into grand rounds, as well as postgraduate and undergraduate seminars, integrates them with other skills being developed in these settings. These strategies are discussed at length in Chapter 7. Important developments to help overcome the limited time and resources include the growing numbers of evidence-based journals and evidence-based summary services. These are discussed throughout the book and in detail in Chapter 2. Indeed, one of the goals of this edition of the book is to provide tips and tools for practicing EBM in "real-time". In addition, we encourage readers to use the website to let us know about ways in which they've managed to meet the challenges of practicing EBM in real-time.

HOW IS THIS PACKAGE (THE BOOK, THE ACCOMPANYING CD, AND THE ASSOCIATED WEBSITE) ORGANIZED?

The overall package is designed to help practitioners from any health care discipline learn how to practice evidence-based health care. Thus, although the book is written within the narrow perspectives of internal medicine and general practice, the CD provides clinical scenarios, questions, searches, critical appraisals, and evidence summaries from other disciplines, permitting readers to apply the strategies and tactics of evidence-based practice to any health discipline.

For those of you who want to become more proficient at being "doers" of EBM, we would suggest that you take a look at Chapters 1–8. For readers who want to become "users" of EBM, we would suggest tackling Chapters 1 and 2, focusing on question formulation and matching those questions to the various evidence resources. We have also provided tips on practicing EBM in real-time throughout the book and on the accompanying CD. Finally, for those interested in teaching the practice of EBM, we have dedicated Chapter 7 to this topic.

The chapters and appendices that comprise this book constitute a traditional way of presenting our ideas about EBM. It offers the "basic" (or "Ka") version of the model for practicing EBM. For those who want more detailed discussion, we would suggest you review some other resources.[36] And, while the examples were current when we wrote this in 2004, by the time this book appears in print, they will be outdated! So, we would suggest that you visit our website (www.cebm.utoronto.ca) for ongoing materials and practice tools. The website can also be used to contact us; in particular, we'd like to hear where we've gone wrong and what we could do better in future editions.

REFERENCES

1   Evidence-Based Medicine Working Group. Evidence-based medicine. A new approach to teaching the practice of medicine. JAMA 1992; 268: 2420–5.

2   Sidorov J. How are internal medicine residency journal clubs organized and what makes them successful? Arch Intern Med 1995; 155: 1193–7.

3   Alguire PC. A review of journal clubs in postgraduate medical education. J Gen Intern Med 1998; 13: 347–53.

4   Hopcroft K. Why the drugs don't work. The Times 13 December, 2003.

5   Osheroff JA, Forsythe DE, Buchanan BG, Bankowitz RA, Blumenfeld BH, Miller RA. Physicians' information needs: analysis of questions posed during clinical teaching. Ann Intern Med 1991; 114: 576–81.

6   Covell DG, Uman GC, Manning PR. Information needs in office practice: are they being met? Ann Intern Med 1985; 103: 596–9.

7   Antman EM, Lau J, Kupelnick B, Mosteller F, Chalmers TC. A comparison of results of meta-analyses of randomised control trials and recommendations of clinical experts. JAMA 1992; 268: 240–8.

8   Oxman A, Guyatt GH. The science of reviewing research. Ann N Y Acad Sci 1993; 703: 125–34.

9   Davis DA, Thomson MA, Oxman AD, Haynes RB. Changing physician performance: a systematic review of the effect of continuing medical education strategies. JAMA 1997; 274: 700–5.

10 Haynes RB. Where's the meat in clinical journals [editorial]? ACP Journal Club 1993; 119: A22–3.

11 Evans CE, Haynes RB, Birkett NJ, et al. Does a mailed continuing education program improve clinician performance? Results of a randomised trial in antihypertensive care. JAMA 1986; 255: 501–4.

12 Sackett DL, Haynes RB, Taylor DW, Gibson ES, Roberts RS, Johnson AL. Clinical determinants of the decision to treat primary hypertension. Clin Res 1977; 24: 648.

13 Sackett DL, Straus SE. Finding and applying evidence during clinical rounds: the "evidence cart". JAMA 1998; 280:1336–8.

14 Sackett DL. Using evidence-based medicine to help physicians keep up-to-date. Serials 1997; 9: 178–81.

15 The Cochrane Library, Issue 1. Update Software, Oxford, 2004.

16 Effective Practice and Organisation of Care Group. The Cochrane Library, Issue 1. Update Software, Oxford, 2004.

17 McAlister FA, Graham I, Karr GW, Laupacis A. Evidence-based medicine and the practicing clinician: a survey of Canadian general internists. J Gen Intern Med 1999; 14: 236–42.

18 McColl A, Smith H, White P, Field J. General practitioners' perceptions of the route to evidence-based medicine: a questionnaire survey. BMJ 1998; 316: 361–5.

19 Young JM, Glasziou P, Ward J. General practitioners' self ratings of skills in evidence based medicine: validation study. BMJ 2002; 324: 950–1.

20 Deshpande N, Publicover M, Gee H, Khan KS. Incorporating the views of obstetric clinicians in implementing evidence-supported labour and delivery suite ward rounds: a case study. Health Info Libr J 2003; 20(2): 86–94.

21 Ellis J, Mulligan I, Rowe J, Sackett D L. Inpatient general medicine is evidence based. Lancet 1995; 346: 407–10.

22 Geddes JR, Game D, Jenkins NE, Peterson LA, Pottinger GR, Sackett DL. In-patient psychiatric care is evidence-based. Proceedings of the Royal College of Psychiatrists Winter Meeting, Stratford, UK, January 23–25, 1996.

23 Howes N, Chagla L, Thorpe M, McCulloch P. Surgical practice is evidence based. Br J Surg 1997; 84: 1220–3.

24 Kenny SE, Shankar KR, Rintala R, Lamont GL, Lloyd DA. Evidence-based surgery: interventions in a regional paediatric surgical unit. Arch Dis Child 1997; 76: 50–3.

25 Gill P, Dowell AC, Neal RD, Smith N, Heywood P, Wilson AE. Evidence based general practice: a retrospective study of interventions in one training practice. BMJ 1996; 312: 819–21.

26 Parkes J, Hyde C, Deeks J, Milne R. Teaching critical appraisal skills in health care settings. Cochrane Library, Issue 1. Update Software, Oxford, 2004.

27 Greenhalgh T, Douglas HR. Experiences of general practitioners and practice nurses of training courses in evidence-based health care: a qualitative study. Br J Gen Pract 1999; 49: 536–40.

28 Rosenberg W, Deeks J, Lusher A, et al. Improving searching skills and evidence retrieval. J R Coll Physicians Lond 1998; 328: 557–63.

29 Straus SE, Ball CM, McAlister FA, et al. Teaching EBM skills can improve practice patterns in a community-based hospital. BMJ (submitted for publication).

30 Mitchell JB, Ballard DJ, Whisnant JP, Ammering CJ, Samsa GP, Matchar DB. What role do neurologists play in determining the costs and outcomes of stroke patients? Stroke 1996; 27: 1937–43.

31 Wong JH, Findlay JM, Suarez-Almazor ME. Regional performance of carotid endarterectomy appropriateness, outcomes and risk factors for complications. Stroke 1997; 28: 891–8.

32 Davis D, Evans M, Jadad A, et al. The case for knowledge translation: shortening the journey from evidence to effect. BMJ 2003; 327: 33–5.

33 Grol R, Grimshaw J. From best evidence to best practice: effective implementation of change in patients' care. Lancet 2003; 362: 1225–30.

34 Straus SE, McAlister FA. Evidence-based medicine: a commentary on common criticisms. Can Med Assoc J 2000; 163: 837–41.

35 Maynard A. Evidence-based medicine: an incomplete method for informing treatment choices. Lancet 1997; 349: 126–8.

36 Guyatt G, Rennie D, eds. Users' Guides to the Medical Literature. Chicago, AMA Press, 2002.

As we noted in the Introduction, as we care for patients we often need new health care knowledge to inform our decisions and actions.[1–3] Our knowledge needs can range from simple, obvious, and readily available to complex, subtle, and much harder to find. While many kinds of knowledge may be useful, often what we need will be evidence derived from clinical care research. In this chapter, we describe strategies for the first step in meeting these evidence needs: asking clinical questions that are answerable from clinical care research. We will start with a patient encounter to remind us how clinical questions arise and to show how they can be used to initiate evidence-based clinical learning. We will also introduce some teaching tactics that can help us coach others to develop their questioning skills.

CLINICAL SCENARIO

You've just begun a month as the attending physician supervising residents and students on a hospital medicine inpatient service. You join the team on rounds after they've finished admitting a patient. The patient is a 76-year-old woman admitted with a history of progressive dyspnea and leg edema. She was diagnosed with congestive heart failure 6 months ago, when she presented with similar complaints, and was found on examination to have elevated neck veins, lung crackles, an S3 gallop, and pitting edema in both legs. On that admission, her ECG showed normal sinus rhythm and her transthoracic echocardiogram showed systolic dysfunction, with an estimated ejection fraction of 25–30%. Since then, she has been treated with diuretics, ACE (angiotensin-converting enzyme) inhibitors, beta-blockers, digoxin, and aspirin and has been hospitalized twice with exacerbations of heart failure. Now, on her third hospitalization, she is frustrated by her continued symptoms and worried about the future, given her frequent exacerbations and admissions to hospital. Her examination shows significant edema, neck vein distension, an S3 gallop, and an abdominal fluid wave. Her ECG shows sinus rhythm, and her chest radiograph shows pulmonary venous congestion with small bilateral effusions.

You ask your team what questions they have about this patient; specifically, what important pieces of medical knowledge they'd like to have in order to provide better care for this patient. What do you expect they would ask? What questions occur to you about this patient? Write the first three of your questions in the boxes below:

1.

2.

3.

The team's medical students asked several questions, including:

a. What can precipitate an acute exacerbation of congestive heart failure?

b. How does congestive heart failure lead to ascites?

c. What did the patient mean by "If my heart has failed, will I flunk, too?"

The team's house officers also asked several questions, including:

a. Among patients presenting with an acute exacerbation of heart failure, how often would a thorough investigation uncover previously unsuspected acute ischemia as the principal (or contributing) precipitant of the episode?

b. In adults with heart failure who are in sinus rhythm, would adding warfarin to standard therapy reduce morbidity or mortality from thromboembolism enough over 3–5 years to be worth the harmful effects and inconveniences of warfarin?

c. In patients with recurrent exacerbations of heart failure, would joining a local, integrated, heart failure disease management program reduce mortality, morbidity, or hospitalizations enough over the next year to be worth the extra time, money, or inconvenience?

BACKGROUND AND FOREGROUND QUESTIONS

Note that the students' questions in the above example concern general knowledge that would help them understand heart failure as a disorder. Such "background" questions can be asked about any disorder or health state, a test, a treatment or intervention, or other aspect of health care, and can encompass biologic, psychologic, or sociologic phenomena.[4] When well formulated, background questions usually have two components (Table 1.1):

Table 1.1 Well-built clinical questions

"Background" questions

- Ask for general knowledge about a condition or thing

- Have two essential components:
  1. A question root (who, what, where, when, how, why), and a verb
  2. A disorder, test, treatment, or other aspect of health care

Examples

"How does heart failure cause ascites?"
"What causes SARS?"

"Foreground" questions

- Ask for specific knowledge to inform clinical decisions or actions

- Have four essential components:

  1. Patient and/or problem
  2. Intervention (or exposure)
  3. Comparison, if relevant
  4. Clinical outcomes, including time if relevant

Example

"In adults with heart failure who are in sinus rhythm, would adding warfarin to standard therapy reduce morbidity or mortality from thromboembolism enough over 3–5 years to be worth warfarin's harmful effects and inconveniences?"

---

1. A question root (who, what, when, where, how, why) with a verb.

2. An aspect of the condition or thing of interest.

Note that the house officers' questions concern specific knowledge that could directly inform one or more "foreground" clinical decisions they face with this patient, including a broad range of biologic, psychologic, and sociologic issues. When well constructed, such foreground questions usually have four components[5,6] (Table 1.1):

1. The patient situation, population, or problem of interest.

2. The main intervention, defined very broadly, including an exposure, a diagnostic test, a prognostic factor, a treatment, a patient perception, and so forth.

3. A comparison intervention or exposure, if relevant.

4. The clinical outcome(s) of interest, including a time horizon if relevant.

Return to the three questions you wrote down about the patient in the example above. Are they background or foreground questions? Do your background questions specify two components (root with verb and condition), and do your foreground questions contain three or four components (patient/problem, intervention, comparison, and outcomes)? If not, try rewriting them to include these components, and consider whether these revised questions come closer to asking what you really want to know.

As clinicians, we all have needs for both background and foreground knowledge, in proportions that vary over time and that depend primarily on our experience with the particular disorder at hand (see Figure 1.1). When our experience with the condition is limited, at point "A" (like a beginning student), the majority of our questions (designated in Figure 1.1 by the vertical dimension) might be about background knowledge. As we grow in clinical experience and responsibility, such as point "B" (like a house officer), we'll have increasing proportions of

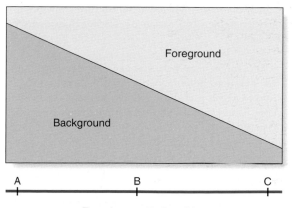

Foreground

Background

A   B   C

Experience with Condition

Figure 1.1 Knowledge needs depend on experience with condition.

questions about the foreground of managing patients. Further experience with the condition puts us at point "C" (like a consultant), where most of our questions will be foreground. Note that the diagonal line is placed to show that we're never too green to learn foreground knowledge, or too experienced to outlive the need for background knowledge.

OUR REACTIONS TO KNOWING AND TO NOT KNOWING

Clinical practice demands that we use large amounts of both background and foreground knowledge, whether or not we're aware of its use. These demands and our awareness come in three combinations, which we will examine here. First, our patient's predicament may call for knowledge we know we already possess, so we will experience the reinforcing mental and emotional responses termed "cognitive resonance" as we apply the knowledge in clinical decisions. Second, we may realize that our patient's illness calls for knowledge we don't possess, and this awareness brings the mental and emotional responses termed "cognitive dissonance" as we confront what we don't know, but need to know. Third, our patient's predicament might call upon knowledge we don't have, yet these gaps may escape our attention, so we don't know what we don't know and we carry on in undisturbed ignorance. (We'll return to this third situation in Chapter 2, where we'll introduce strategies to regularly strengthen and update our knowledge of current best evidence.)

Reflect for a moment on how you've learned to react to the first two situations noted above. When teachers asked questions to which you knew the answers, did you learn to raise your hand to be called upon to give the answers out loud? We did, as did virtually all of our learners, and in the process we've learned that teachers and examinations reward us for knowing already. When teachers asked questions to which you didn't know the answers, did you learn to raise your hand to be called upon and say "I don't know this, but I can see how useful it would be to know and I'm ready to learn it today"? Didn't think so, and neither did we or our learners, so in the process we've all learned that teachers and examinations do not reward us for showing our ignorance and being ready and willing to learn.

Situations of cognitive dissonance (we know that we don't know) can become powerful motivators for learning, if handled well, such as by celebrating the finding of knowledge needs and by turning the "negative space" of knowledge gaps into the "positive space" of well-built clinical questions and learning how to find the answers.[7,8] Unfortunately, if handled less well, our cognitive dissonance might lead us to less adaptive behaviors, such as trying to hide our deficits, or by reacting with anger, fear, or shame.[9] By developing awareness of our knowing and thinking, we can recognize our cognitive dissonance when it occurs, recognize when the knowledge we need would come from clinical care research, and articulate the background or foreground questions we can use to find the answers.

WHERE AND HOW CLINICAL QUESTIONS ARISE

As you might expect, over the years we've found that most of our foreground questions arise around the central issues involved in caring for patients (see Table 1.2). These groupings are neither jointly exhaustive (other worthwhile questions can be asked), nor mutually exclusive (some questions are hybrids, asking about both prognosis and therapy for example). Still, we find it useful to anticipate that many of our questions will arise from common locations on this "map": clinical findings, etiology, differential diagnosis, diagnostic tests, prognosis, therapy, prevention, patient experience and meaning, and self-improvement. We keep this list handy and use it to help locate the source of our knowledge deficits when we recognize the "stuck" feelings of our cognitive dissonance. Once we've recognized our knowledge gaps, articulating the questions can be done quickly, usually in 30 seconds or less.

Over the years we've found that many of our knowledge needs occur around, or even during, our clinical encounters with patients. While often they arise first in our heads, just as often they are voiced at least in part by our patients themselves. For instance, when a patient asks "What is the matter?" this relates to questions about diagnosis that arise in our minds. Similarly, "What will this mean for me?" conjures both prognosis, and experience and meaning questions, while "What should be done?" brings up issues of treatment and prevention. No matter who initiates the questions, we consider finding relevant answers as one of the ways we serve our patients, and to indicate this responsibility we call these questions ours. When we can manage to do so, we find it helpful to negotiate explicitly with our patients about which questions should be addressed, in what order, and by when. And, increasingly often we're discovering that patients want to work on answering some of these questions with us.

Table 1.2 Central issues in clinical work, where clinical questions often arise

1. **Clinical findings**: how to properly gather and interpret findings from the history and physical examination.

2. **Etiology**: how to identify causes or risk factors for disease (including iatrogenic harms).

3. **Clinical manifestations of disease**: knowing how often and when a disease causes its clinical manifestations and how to use this knowledge in classifying our patients' illnesses.

4. **Differential diagnosis**: when considering the possible causes of our patient's clinical problems, how to select those that are likely, serious, and responsive to treatment.

5. **Diagnostic tests**: how to select and interpret diagnostic tests, in order to confirm or exclude a diagnosis, based on considering their precision, accuracy, acceptability, safety, expense, etc.

6. **Prognosis**: how to estimate our patient's likely clinical course over time and anticipate likely complications of the disorder.

7. **Therapy**: how to select treatments to offer our patients that do more good than harm and that are worth the efforts and costs of using them.

8. **Prevention**: how to reduce the chance of disease by identifying and modifying risk factors and how to diagnose disease early by screening.

9. **Experience and meaning**: how to empathize with our patients' situations, appreciate the meaning they find in the experience, and understand how this meaning influences their healing.

10. **Improvement**: how to keep up-to-date, improve our clinical and other skills, and run a better, more efficient, clinical care system.

SELECTING, SCHEDULING, AND SAVING QUESTIONS TO ANSWER

Since our patients' illness burdens are large and our available time is small, we find that we usually have many more questions than time in which to answer them. For this circumstance, we recommend three strategies: selecting, scheduling, and saving.

First, by "selecting" we mean deciding which one or few of the many questions we asked should be pursued. This decision requires judgment and we'd suggest you consider the nature of the patient's illness, the nature of your knowledge needs, the specific clinical decisions in which you'll use the knowledge, and your role in that decision process. Then, try this sequence of filters:

1. Which question is most important to the patient's well-being, whether biologic, psychologic, or sociologic?

2. Which question is most relevant to your/your learners' knowledge needs?

3. Which question is most feasible to answer within the time you have available?

4. Which question is most interesting to you, your learners, or your patient?

5. Which question is most likely to recur in your practice?

With a moment of reflection, you can usually select one or two questions that best pass these tests and will best inform the decisions at hand.

Second, by "scheduling" we mean deciding by when we need to have our questions answered, paying particular attention to when the resulting decisions need to be made. While integrated clinical care and information systems may improve to the point at which our questions will be answerable at the time they arise, for most of us this is not yet the case, and we need to be realistic in planning our time. With a moment of reflection, you can usually discern the few questions that demand immediate answers from the majority that can be answered later that day or at the next scheduled appointment.

The third strategy involves "saving" our questions. Since it seems obvious that unsaved questions become unanswered questions, it follows that we need practical methods to rapidly record questions for later retrieval and searching. Having just encouraged you to articulate your questions fully, it may surprise you that we recommend using very brief notations when recording questions on the run, using shorthand that makes sense to you. For instance, when we jot down "wt loss CMD depression," we mean "Among adults confirmed to have major depressive disorder who undergo thorough evaluation, what proportion will have unexplained weight loss as their principal presenting problem?" (a question of the frequency of clinical manifestations of disease, hence "CMD").

But how best to record these questions? Over the years, we've tried, or heard of others trying, several solutions:

1. Jotting brief notes on a page with four columns drawn, one for each of the elements of foreground questions.

2. Keying brief notes into a similarly arrayed electronic file on a desktop computer.

3. Dictating questions into a pocket-sized recording device.

4. Jotting concise questions onto actual prescription blanks (and remembering not to give them to the patient instead of their actual prescriptions!).

5. Jotting shorthand notes onto 3×5 cards kept in a handy pocket.

6. Turning on a PDA and tapping in similar shorthand notes.

Whenever we've timed ourselves, we find it takes us about 15 seconds to record the gist of our questions.[10]

PRACTICING EBM IN REAL-TIME

Recording, storing, and retrieving our questions can be significant challenges. Several colleagues have developed software that we can use on our PDAs that help us develop and save our questions. For example, with PICOmaker (www.library.ualberta.ca/pdazone/pico/), we can save questions to our PalmPilots. We've provided another example of a clinical question on the accompanying CD that you can download to your PDA. Once installed, these programs sit in your pocket, waiting to guide you through the steps of formulating questions and saving them for later retrieval.

WHY BOTHER FORMULATING QUESTIONS CLEARLY?

Our own experiences suggest that well-formulated questions can help in seven ways:

1. They help us focus our scarce learning time on evidence that is directly relevant to our patients' clinical needs.

2. They help us focus our scarce learning time on evidence that directly addresses our particular knowledge needs, or those of our learners.

3. They can suggest high-yield search strategies (see Ch. 2).

4. They suggest the forms that useful answers might take (see Chs 3–6).

5. When sending or receiving a patient in referral, they can help us to communicate more clearly with our colleagues.

6. When teaching, they can help our learners to better understand the content of what we teach, while also modeling some adaptive processes for lifelong learning.

7. When our questions get answered, our knowledge grows, our curiosity is reinforced, our cognitive resonance is restored, and we can become better, faster, and happier clinicians.

In addition, the research we've seen so far suggests that clinicians who are taught this structured approach ask more specific questions,[11] undertake more searches for evidence,[12] use more detailed search methods and find more precise answers.[13,14] Also, if when family doctors "curbside consult" their specialty colleagues they include a clinical question that is clearly articulated along these lines, they are more likely to receive an answer.[15] Some groups have begun to implement and evaluate question-answering services for their clinicians, with similarly promising initial results.[16,17]

Tm

TEACHING THE ASKING OF ANSWERABLE CLINICAL QUESTIONS

Good questions are the backbone of both practicing and teaching EBM, and patients serve as the starting point for both. Our challenge as teachers is to identify questions that are both patient-based (arising out of the clinical problems of this real patient under the learner's care) and learner-centered (targeting the learning needs of this learner). As we become more skilled at asking questions ourselves, we should also become more skilled in teaching others how to do so.

As with other clinical skills, most of us teach question-asking best by modeling the formation of good clinical questions in front of our learners. We can also model admitting that we don't know it all, identifying our own knowledge gaps, and showing our learners adaptive ways of responding to the resulting cognitive dissonance. Once we've modeled asking a few questions, we can stop and describe explicitly what we did, noting each of the elements of good questions, whether background or foreground.

The four main steps in teaching clinical learners how to ask good questions are listed in Table 1.3. If we are to recognize potential questions in learners' cases, help them select the "best" question to focus on, guide them in building that question well, and assess their question-building performance and skill, we need to be proficient at building questions ourselves. Moreover, we need several attributes of good clinical teaching, such as good listening skills, enthusiasm, and a willingness to help learners develop to

Table 1.3 Key steps in teaching how to ask questions for EBM
1. **Recognize**: how to identify combinations of a patient's needs and a learner's needs that represent opportunities for the learner to build good questions.
2. **Select**: how to select from the recognized opportunities the one (or few) that best fits the needs of the patient and the learner at that clinical moment.
3. **Guide**: how to guide the learner in transforming knowledge gaps into well-built clinical questions.
4. **Assess**: how to assess the learner's performance and skill at asking pertinent, answerable clinical questions for practicing EBM.

their full potential. It helps to be able to spot signs of our learners' cognitive dissonance, to know when and what they're ready to learn.

Note that teaching question-asking skills can be integrated with any other clinical teaching, right at the bedside or other site of patient care, and it needn't take much additional time. Modeling question formulation takes less than a minute, while coaching learners on asking a question about a patient usually takes 2–3 minutes.

Once we have formulated an important question with our learners, how might we keep track of it and follow its progress toward a clinically useful answer? In addition to the methods for saving questions we mentioned earlier, one tactic we've used for teaching question formulation is the "educational prescription", shown in Figure 1.2. These help both teachers and learners in five ways:

1. It specifies the clinical problem that generated the questions.

2. It states the question, in all of its key elements.

3. It specifies who is responsible for answering it.

4. It reminds everyone of the deadline for answering it (taking into account the urgency of the clinical problem that generated it).

R Educational Prescription

| Patient's Name | Learner: |

3-part Clinical Question

Target Disorder:

Intervention (+/− comparison):

Outcome:

Date and place to be filled:

Presentations will cover:
1. search strategy;
2. search results;
3. the validity of this evidence;
4. the importance of this valid evidence;
5. can this valid, important evidence be applied to your patient;
6. your evaluation of this process.

Figure 1.2 Educational prescription form.

5. Finally, it reminds everyone of the steps of searching, critically appraising, and relating the answer back to the patient.

How might we use the educational prescription in our clinical teaching? The number of ways is limited only by our imaginations and our opportunities for teaching. As we'll reinforce in Chapter 7, educational prescriptions have been incorporated into familiar inpatient teaching settings from work rounds and attending/consultant rounds to morning report and noon conferences. They have also been used in outpatient teaching settings, such as ambulatory morning report. You can download these forms from the accompanying CD and website.

Will you and your learners follow through on the educational prescriptions? You might, if you build the writing and "dispensing" of them into your everyday routine. One tactic we use is to make specifying clinical questions an integral part of presenting a new patient to the group. For example, we ask learners on our general medicine inpatient clinical teams, when presenting new patients, to tell us "33 things in 3 minutes" about each admission, although only the first 25 at the bedside. As shown in Table 1.4, the final element of their presentation is the specification of an important question to which they need to know the answer and don't. If the answer is vital to the immediate care of the patient, it can be provided at once by another member of the clinical team, perhaps by accessing some of the evidence synopsis resources you'll learn more about in Chapter 2. Most of the time the answer can wait a few hours or days, so the question can serve as the start of an educational prescription.

Finally, we can ask our learners to write educational prescriptions for us. This role reversal can help in four ways:

1. The learners must supervise our question-building, thereby honing their skills further.

2. The learners see us admitting our own knowledge gaps and practicing what we preach.

3. It adds fun to rounds and sustains group morale.

4. Our learners begin to prepare for their later roles as clinical teachers.

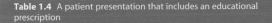

Table 1.4 A patient presentation that includes an educational prescription

1. The patient's surname.
2. The patient's age.
3. The patient's gender (if NOT presenting at the bedside).
4. When the patient was admitted.
5. The chief complaint(s) that led to admission. For each complaint, mention the following:
    6. Where in the body it is located.
    7. Its quality.
    8. Its quantity, intensity, and degree of impairment.
    9. Its chronology: when it began, constant/episodic, progressive.
    10. Its setting: under what circumstances did/does it occur.
    11. Any aggravating or alleviating factors.
    12. Any associated symptoms.
13. Whether a similar complaint had happened previously. If so:
    14. How it was investigated.
    15. What the patient was told about its cause.
    16. How the patient had been treated for it.
17. Pertinent past history of other conditions that are of diagnostic, prognostic or pragmatic significance, and would affect the evaluation or treatment of the chief complaint.
18. And how those other conditions have been treated.
19. Family history, if pertinent to chief complaint or hospital care.
20. Social history, if pertinent to chief complaint or hospital care.

21. The patient's:
    a. Ideas (What they think is wrong with them).
    b. Concerns (What they are worried about).
    c. Expectations (What is going to happen to and for them).
22. The condition on admission:
    a. Acutely and/or chronically ill.
    b. Severity of complaints.
    c. Requesting what sort of help.
23. The pertinent physical findings on admission.
24. The pertinent diagnostic test results.
25. Your concise, one-sentence problem synthesis statement.

Table 1.4 *(cont'd)*

And, if NOT presenting at the bedside:

26. What you think the most likely diagnosis is ("leading hypothesis").

27. What few other diagnoses you're pursuing ("active alternatives").

28. The further diagnostic studies you plan to confirm the leading hypothesis or exclude active alternatives.

29. Your estimate of the patient's prognosis.

30. Your plans for treatment and counseling.

31. How you will monitor the treatment in follow-up.

32. Your contingency plans if the patient doesn't respond to treatment.

33. The educational prescription you would like to write for yourself in order to better understand the patient's disorder (background knowledge), or how to care for the patient (foreground knowledge) in order to become a better clinician.

That concludes this chapter on the first step in practicing and teaching EBM: asking answerable clinical questions. Since you and your learners will want to move quickly from asking questions to finding their answers, our next chapter will address this second step in practicing and teaching EBM.

REFERENCES

1 Smith R. What clinical information do doctors need? BMJ 1996; 313: 1062–8.

2 Dawes M, Sampson U. Knowledge management in clinical practice: a systematic review of information seeking behavior in physicians. Int J Med Inf 2003; 71: 9–15.

3 Case DO. Looking for Information: A Survey of Research on Information Seeking, Needs, and Behavior. San Diego, CA: Academic Press, 2002.

4 Richardson WS. Ask, and ye shall retrieve [EBM note]. Evidence-Based Medicine 1998; 3:100–1.

5 Oxman AD, Sackett DL, Guyatt GH, for the Evidence-Based Medicine Working Group. Users' guides to the medical literature. I. How to get started. JAMA 1993; 270: 2093–5.

6 Richardson WS, Wilson MC, Nishikawa J, Hayward RSA. The well-built clinical question: a key to evidence-based decisions [editorial]. ACP J Club 1995; 123: A12–A13.

7 Neighbour R. The Inner Apprentice: An Awareness-Centred Approach to Vocational Training for General Practice. Newbury, UK: Petroc Press, 1996.

8 Schon DA. Educating the Reflective Practitioner. San Francisco, CA: Jossey-Bass, 1987.

9 Claxton G. Wise-Up: The Challenge of Lifelong Learning. New York, NY: Bloomsbury, 1999.

10 Richardson WS, Burdette SD. Practice corner: taking evidence in hand [editorial]. ACP J Club 2003; 138: A9–A10.

11   Villanueva EV, Burrows EA, Fennessy PA, Rajendran M, Anderson JN. Improving question formulation for use in evidence appraisal in a tertiary care setting: a randomised controlled trial. BMC Med Inf Decis Making 2001; I: 4.

12   Cabell CH, Schardt C, Sanders L, Corey GR, Keitz SA. Resident utilization of information technology. J Gen Intern Med 2001; 16: 838–44.

13   Booth A, O'Rourke AJ, Ford NJ. Structuring the pre-search interview: a useful technique for handling clinical questions. Bull Med Libr Assoc 2000; 88: 239–46.

14   Rosenberg WM, Deeks J, Lusher A, Snowball R, Dooley G, Sackett D. Improving searching skills and evidence retrieval. J R Coll Phys London 1998; 32: 557–63.

15   Bergus GR, Randall CS, Sinift SD, Rosenthal DM. Does the structure of clinical questions affect the outcome of curbside consultations with specialty colleagues? Arch Fam Med 2000; 9: 541–7.

16   Brassey J, Elwyn G, Price C, Kinnersley P. Just in time information for clinicians: a questionnaire evaluation of the ATTRACT project. BMJ 2001; 322: 529–30.

17   Jerome RN, Giuse NB, Gish KW, Sathe NA, Dietrich MS. Information needs of clinical teams: analysis of questions received by the Clinical Informatics Consult Service. Bull Med Libr Assoc 2001; 89: 177–84.

How to find current best evidence

and have current best evidence find us

My students are dismayed when I say to them "Half of what you are taught as medical students will in 10 years have been shown to be wrong. And the trouble is, none of your teachers knows which half."

(Dr Sydney Burwell, Dean of Harvard Medical School[1])

As highlighted in the Preface, keeping up-to-date with current best evidence for the care of our patients is challenging. As Dr Burwell's quote from half a century ago indicates, new medical knowledge was evolving quite quickly then. In the past decade, the pace has accelerated because of the maturation of biomedical research (from bench to bedside), and huge new investments in health care research of over US$100 billion per year.

One solution for the problem of obsolescence of professional education is "problem-based learning" or "learning by inquiry". That is, when confronted by a clinical question for which we are unsure of the current best answer, we need to develop the habit of looking for the current best answer as efficiently as possible. (Literary critics will point out the redundancy of the term "current best"—we risk their scorn to emphasize that last year's best answer may not be this year's.)

The success of learning by inquiry depends heavily on being able to find the current best evidence to manage pressing clinical problems, a task that can be either quick and highly rewarding or time-consuming and frustrating. Which of these it is depends on several factors that we can control or influence, including which questions we ask, how we ask these questions (see Ch. 1), which information resources we use (the subject of this chapter), and how skilled we are in interpreting and applying these resources (detailed in the chapters that follow). We can learn a great deal about current best information sources from librarians and other experts in medical informatics, and should seek hands-on training from them as an essential part of our clinical training. This chapter provides adjunctive searching strategies for clinicians to use to find evidence quickly—including some that you may not learn from librarians—as well as an approach to dealing with evidence that finds us, bidden or unbidden.

Here, we consider finding evidence to help solve clinical problems about the treatment or prevention, diagnosis and differential diagnosis, prognosis and clinical prediction, cause, and economics of a clinical problem. "Best-evidence" resources are built according to an explicit process that values research according to its scientific merit ("hierarchy of research methods") and clinical relevance. You will learn these principles as you go through this book. To be useful for providing the evidence we need for a particular clinical problem, best-evidence resources must be in formats that facilitate rapid searching to find exact matches for clinical questions. Whether the search engine is electronic or manual (e.g. scanning the pages of a pocket notebook), the important features are portability and easy navigation from clinical questions to evidence-based answers. Fortunately for the readers of this book, this combination of evidence-based content and easy access is now available for a rapidly growing number of health care problems, with vigorous efforts underway to tackle clinical disciplines that are presently not well served. The next part of this chapter provides an orientation to the types of evidence-based sources that exist today. This is followed by opportunities to track down the answers to specific clinical problems.

ORIENTATION TO EVIDENCE-BASED INFORMATION RESOURCES
Where to find the best evidence
1. *Burn your traditional textbooks*
We begin with textbooks, only to dismiss all but the best of a new breed of them. If the pages of textbooks smelled like decomposing garbage when they are outdated, the non-smelly bits could be useful, because textbooks are generally

well organized for clinical use and much of their content will be current at any one time. Unfortunately, in most texts, there's no way to tell what is up-to-date and what is not. So, although we may find some useful information in texts about "background questions", such as the pathophysiology of clinical problems, it is best not to use them for seeking the answers to "foreground questions", such as the causal (risk) factors, diagnosis, prognosis, prevention or treatment of a disorder if there is an up-to-date, evidence-based alternative.

About now, you might be asking if we really mean that you should burn your traditional textbooks. We do. At this point, our publisher is probably getting edgy about where this discussion is heading, considering all the journals and textbooks they publish, including this one. Any money saved from purchasing traditional textbooks can be well spent on better sources of current best knowledge for clinical practice. If the direction we've taken so far makes you tense, please relax and enjoy the rest of this trip, which is heading into the "4S" territory of evidence-based resources.

2. Take a "4S" approach to evidence-based information access*

Practical resources to support evidence-based health care decisions are rapidly evolving. New and better services are being created through the combined forces of increasing numbers of clinically important studies, more robust evidence synthesis and synopsis services, and better information technology and systems. You can help yourself to best current evidence by recognizing and using the most evolved information services for the topics that interest you.

Figure 2.1 provides a 4S hierarchical structure, with original "studies" at the base, "syntheses" (systematic reviews) of evidence just above the base, followed by "synopses" of studies and syntheses, and, finally, the most evolved evidence-based information "systems" at the top. *You should*

---

* With permission from the American College of Physicians, this section draws heavily on: Haynes RB. Of studies, summaries, synopses, and systems: the 4S evolution of services for finding current best evidence [editorial]. ACP J Club 2001; 134: A11–3 (Evid Based Med 2001; 6: 36–8).

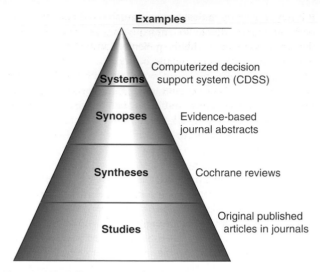

Examples

Systems — Computerized decision support system (CDSS)

Synopses — Evidence-based journal abstracts

Syntheses — Cochrane reviews

Studies — Original published articles in journals

Figure 2.1 The "4S" organization of evidence from research.

begin your search for best evidence by looking at the highest-level resource available for the problem that prompts your search. The details of how to do this follow.

Systems

The ideal. A perfect evidence-based clinical information *system* would integrate and concisely summarize all relevant and important research evidence about a clinical problem and would automatically link, through an electronic medical record, a specific patient's circumstances to the relevant information. We would then consult—indeed, be prompted by—the system whenever the patient's medical record is reviewed. The information contained in the system would be based on an explicit review process for finding and evaluating new evidence as it is published and then reliably and promptly updated whenever important new research evidence becomes available. The clinician and patient could therefore always have the benefit of the current best evidence.

It is important to note that such a system would not tell decision-makers what to do. These judgments need to integrate the system's evidence with the patient's circumstances and wishes.[2] The system's role would be to ensure that the cumulative research evidence concerning the patient's problem is immediately at hand. Further, to maximize speed of use, our first point of interaction would be a short *synopsis*, but links to *syntheses* and then to original *studies* would be provided so that we could drill down as deeply as needed to verify the accuracy, currency, and details of the synopsis.

The present state of evolution. Current systems don't reach this level of perfection as yet, but production models exist for parts of such systems. Electronic medical record systems with computerized decision support rules have been shown in randomized trials to improve the process and sometimes the outcome of care.[3] However, these systems cover a limited range of clinical problems, are not necessarily based on current best evidence, and are mainly "homebuilt" and thus are not easily transferred to most practice settings.

Given that we have some way to go before current best evidence is integrated into electronic medical records, some excellent, but less-developed, systems are readily available. *Clinical Evidence* from the BMJ Publishing Group is the current pace-setter (http://www.clinicalevidence.com*, and as a separate title in Ovid†). At present, *Clinical Evidence* includes only evidence for treatment of a relatively limited but expanding range of clinical questions. The American College of Physicians (ACP) provides PIER (the *Physician's Information and Education Resource*); this is an evidence-based on-line text for ACP members (http://pier.acponline.org /index.html), with explicit grading of evidence for internal medicine and primary care. *UpToDate*,[4] on CD and the web (http://www.uptodate.com), is updated quarterly,

---

* In the wild world of the Internet, URLs often change. If this or any other URL in the book doesn't work, "google" the title of the publication (go to www.google.com and put the title in the search line) and you will likely find the new URL.

† Ask your librarian. Ovid serves many hospital and university libraries, but your library may or may not subscribe to *Clinical Evidence* this way. If not, politely request that it does so.

extensively referenced, and provides MEDLINE abstracts for key evidence. This provides the user at least a sporting chance of dating and appraising the supporting evidence. *ACP Medicine* (formerly *Scientific American Medicine*[5]) also extensively references its contents, and its Internet version (http://www.acpmedicine.com/) is augmented with links to MEDLINE citations and abstracts, as well as many other web resources. *Harrison's Principles of Internal Medicine*,[6] available in several formats (http://www.harrisonsmed.com/), has been upgrading its currency and provides more references and abstracts on its web version, although the extent of referencing is still very limited, and much of the text is updated only once in 3 years. More specialized clinical content is provided in such offerings as *Evidence Based on Call* (http://www.eboncall.org/content.jsp.htm), *Evidence Based Pediatrics and Child Health* (http://www.evidbasedpediatrics.com/), and *Evidence Based Cardiology* (http://www.evidbasedcardiology.com/).

We look forward to many more such texts soon; but beware, these texts are in transition. It is important to check whether the systematic consideration of evidence promised in the title and introduction of these books is actually delivered in the contents. Unfortunately, the term "evidence-based" has been adopted by many publishers and authors without the savvy or scruples to deliver honest evidence-based content. Thus, your first task in seeking evidence-based systems is to look for texts and websites that:

- Are revised at least once a year: each chapter or section should have a date of most recent revision.

- Select and appraise evidence in an explicit way: the introductory section of the text should give a blow-by-blow, reproducible description of the procedure used.

- Cite evidence in support of declarations about clinical care: readers can thus get to original sources for details and can also easily determine the date of publication of evidence cited to support a given claim.

Although none of the systems described above are integrated with electronic medical records, they can be run through the same computers that run electronic medical records so that one need not go to a remote location to find them. Even when best evidence from research is immediately juxtaposed to the clinical record, however, connecting the right information to a specific patient's problems requires that we understand evidence-based care principles and that we apply skill and judgment in using the resources. Fortunately, these emerging information systems reduce these burdens considerably.

Internet-based "aggregators" provide a special "4S supermarket" service in providing access to evidence-based information. Ovid, for example, provides access to a huge collection of texts, journals, and databases, including systems such as *Clinical Evidence*. Ovid's *Evidence Based Medicine Reviews* (EBMR) takes this several steps further in providing access to the Cochrane Library, *ACP Journal Club*, the *Database of Abstracts of Reviews of Evidence* (DARE), and MEDLINE, all in an integrated format that permits tracking from, for example, a full-text original article to a synopsis that describes it, a synthesis (systematic review) in which it is incorporated, and related articles on the same topic.

The systems mentioned here are but a few of those available today. If your discipline or clinical question isn't mentioned in this chapter, consult the more complete listing in the accompanying CD, or try SCHARR (http://www.shef. ac.uk/~scharr/ir/netting/) or Google (www.google.com; put "evidence-based" followed by your discipline on Google's search line).

Synopses

When no evidence-based information system exists for a clinical problem, then *synopses* of individual studies and reviews are the next best source. What busy practitioner has time to use evidence-based resources if the evidence is presented in its original form or even as detailed systematic reviews? Although these detailed articles and reviews are essential building blocks, they are often too heavy to lift on the run. The perfect synopsis of a review or original study would provide only, and exactly, enough information to support a clinical action. The declarative title for each abstract that appears in *ACP Journal Club* and *Evidence Based Medicine* (we'll describe these evidence-based journals later in this chapter) represents an attempt at this. For example, "Review: low-molecular-weight heparin is effective and safe in the acute coronary syndromes". In some circumstances, this title provides enough information to allow the decision-maker either to proceed, assuming familiarity with the nature of the intervention and its alternatives, or to look further for the details, which, for an ideal synopsis, are immediately at hand. The full abstract for this item is in *ACP Journal Club*, with an abstract and commentary on one page,[7] accessible in the original print issue or electronically. Electronic access is definitely the best way to go for all these resources (more about that later).

Syntheses

If more detail is needed or no synopsis is at hand, then databases of systematic reviews (*syntheses*) are available, notably the Cochrane Library, which is available on a quarterly CD, the Internet (http://www.cochranelibrary. com/), and Ovid's EBMR service. These summaries are based on exhaustive searches for evidence, explicit scientific reviews of the studies uncovered in the search, and systematic assembly of the evidence, to provide as clear a signal about the effects of a health care intervention as the accumulated evidence will allow. The *Cochrane Reviews* have focused on preventive or therapeutic interventions to date, but the Cochrane Collaboration recently gave its blessing to reviewers interested in summarizing diagnostic test evidence.

Stimulated by the success of the Cochrane Collaboration, the number of systematic reviews in the medical literature has grown tremendously in the past few years; if the Cochrane Library doesn't have a review on the topic you are interested in, it is worthwhile looking in MEDLINE. Better still, Ovid's EBMR provides one-stop shopping for both Cochrane and non-Cochrane systematic reviews. For the example of low molecular weight heparin for acute coronary syndromes, a search on Ovid's integrated collection of *ACP Journal Club, Cochrane Database of Systematic Reviews* (CDSR), and DARE, using the terms "acute coronary syndromes" and "low molecular weight heparins", retrieved seven items, including a recently updated *Cochrane Review* (synthesis) and three related *ACP Journal Club* items (synopses).

Studies

It takes time to summarize new evidence, and systems, synopses and syntheses necessarily follow the publication of original *studies*, usually by at least 6 months, and sometimes by years. If every other "S" fails (i.e. no systems, synopses, or syntheses exist with clear answers to your question), then it's time to look for original studies. Looking for these in full-text print journals, as we've seen, is generally hopeless, but studies can be retrieved relatively efficiently on the Internet in several ways. If you don't know which database is best suited to your question, "meta" search engines tuned for health care content can assemble access across a number of web-based services. At least one of these search engines is attentive to issues of quality of evidence: namely, SUMSearch (http://sumsearch. uthscsa.edu/). Nevertheless, we must appraise the items identified by such a search to determine which fall within the schema presented here. Many of the items will not, especially when convenience of access is favored over quality.

There are also at least two levels of evidence-based databases to search directly: specialized and general. If the topic falls within the areas of internal medicine, primary care, nursing or mental health, then *ACP Journal Club* (www.acpjc.org, formerly *Best Evidence*), *Evidence Based Medicine* (http://ebm. bmjjournals.com/), *Evidence Based Nursing* (http:// ebn.bmjjournals.com/), and *Evidence Based Mental Health* (http://ebmh.bmjjournals.com/), respectively, provide specialized, evidence-based services because the abstracted articles have been appraised for scientific merit and clinical relevance. If the search is for a treatment, then the Cochrane Library includes the Cochrane Central Register of Controlled

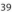

Trials, also available as part of EBMR on Ovid, where it is integrated with *ACP Journal Club* and DARE. But all these services are subject to the timeline required for evidence summarization, to which is added the Ovid timeline for electronic posting and integration.

For original articles and reviews hot off the press, MEDLINE itself is freely available (http://www.ncbi.nlm.nih.gov/ PubMed/), and the Clinical Queries screen (available as a menu item on the main PubMed screen or directly at http://www.ncbi.nlm.nih.gov/entrez/query/static/clinical. html) provides detailed search strategies that home in on clinical content for therapy, diagnosis, prognosis, clinical prediction, etiology, economics, and systematic reviews. These search strategies have recently been upgraded and are embedded in the Clinical Queries screen, so that you don't need to remember them. You can use the "sensitive" search strategy if you want to retrieve every article that might bear on your question. Or you can use the "specific" search strategy if you want "a few good references" and don't have time to sort out the citations that aren't on target.

These search strategies can also be run in proprietary systems that include the MEDLINE database, although they need some translation for the search syntax that is unique to each system. A summary of the best strategies appears in Table 2.1, optimized for Ovid's search engine.

If you still have no luck and the topic is, say, a new treatment (that one of your patients has asked about but you don't yet know about . . .), then you can try Google (http://www.google. com). It is incredibly fast and you can retrieve a product monograph in a few milliseconds in which you'll find what the manufacturer of the treatment claims it can do along with detailed information on adverse effects, contraindications, and prescribing. The Google home page allows you to add a Google search window to your web browser's tool bar. Google is the fastest way to get to almost any service on the Internet that you haven't "bookmarked" for your web browser, including all the ones named in this article that are web-accessible.

Table 2.1 Search strategies for clinical evidence retrieval from MEDLINE in Ovid

Strategy type	Ovid strategy	Sensitivity (%)	Specificity (%)
Therapy			
High sensitivity	clinical trial.mp. OR clinical trial. pt. OR random:. mp. OR tu.xs	99	70
High specificity	randomized controlled trial. pt. OR randomi-zed controlled trial.mp.	93	97
Optimal balance	randomized controlled trial.pt. OR randomized. mp. OR placebo. mp.	96	95
Diagnosis			
High sensitivity	sensitiv:.mp. OR diagnos:.mp. OR di.fs.	98	74
High specificity	specificity.tw.	64	98
Optimal balance	sensitiv:.mp. OR predictive value:. mp. OR accurac:. tw.	93	92
Prognosis			
High sensitivity	incidence.sh. OR exp mortality OR follow-up studies. sh. OR mortality. sh. OR prognos:. tw. OR predict:.tw. OR course:.tw.	90	80
High specificity	prognos:.tw. OR first episode.tw. OR cohort.tw.	52	94
Optimal balance	prognosis.sh. OR diagnosed.tw. OR cohort:.mp. OR predictor:.tw. OR death.tw. OR exp models, statistical	83	84

Table 2.1 *(cont'd)*

Strategy type	Ovid strategy	Sensitivity (%)	Specificity (%)
Clinical prediction guides			
High sensitivity	predict:.mp. OR scor:.tw. OR observ:mp.	96	79
High specificity	validation.tw. OR validate.tw.	54	99
Optimal balance	predict:tw. OR validat:.mp. OR develop.tw.	90	90
Reviews			
High sensitivity	review.pt. OR meta analysis.mp,pt. OR tu.xs.	98	69
High specificity	search strategy.tw.	59	99.9
Optimal balance	review.pt. OR meta-analys:.tw. OR cochrane.tw.	93	92

To use these strategies in Ovid, include the clinical topic terms for your search as one line, type the appropriate strategy from the table on a second line, then put "1 AND 2" on the third line.

3. Organize access to evidence-based information services

It's worth emphasizing that almost all the resources just reviewed are available on the Internet. The added value of accessing these services on the Internet is considerable, including links to full-text journal articles, patient information, and complementary texts. To be able to do this, you need to be in a location, such as a medical library, hospital or clinic, where all the necessary licenses have been obtained, or, better still, have proxy server permission from whatever organizations you belong to, whether it be a university, hospital or professional corporation, so that you can use these services wherever you plug your computer into the Internet. A typical package of services for health professionals might include an Ovid collection of full-text journals, EBMR, *Clinical Evidence* and *ACP Medicine*, plus MD Consult, Stat!Ref, and a separate license for *UpToDate*.

You should ask your university, professional school, hospital, or clinic librarian about what digital library licenses are available and how you can tap into them. If you lack local institutional access, you may still be in luck, depending on the region you live in. For example, the UK National Health Service provides a broad range of evidence-based and other information to all health professionals and citizens through its National Electronic Library of Health (NeLH, http://www.nelh.nhs.uk/), and Australia and Latin-American countries have free access to the Cochrane Library. Also, many professional societies provide access to some of the resources at reduced rates.

Don't assume that your institution or professional society will make evidence-based choices about the publications and services it provides. You should decide which services you need for your clinical work and then check to see if these have been chosen by your institution. If not, make a case for the resources you want. When you do so, be prepared to indicate what your library could give up. Library budgeting is a zero-sum game at best these days. The easiest targets for discontinuation are high-priced, low-impact-factor journals, and it will be perceived as a whole lot less self-serving if you target publications in your own clinical discipline that are at the bottom end of the evidence-based ladder of evolution, rather than the high-priced favorite journals of your colleagues in other disciplines.

If you live in a country with low resources, don't despair! The Health Internetwork Access to Research Information program (HINARI, http://www.healthInternetwork.net/) provides institutional access to a wide range of journals and texts at no or low cost.

If you are on your own, have no computer, can't afford to subscribe to journals, but have access to a public library with a computer linked to the Internet, you're still in luck. Free access to high-quality evidence-based information abounds on the Internet; beginning with PubMed and its full-text links; open-access journals, such as BioMed Central (http://www.biomedcentral.com/), and the Public

Library of Science (http://www.publiclibraryofscience.org/); the many evidence-based resources available through SCHARR (http://www.shef.ac.uk/~scharr/ir/netting/); and the CD listings in this book. Beware, however, that using free Internet services requires a commitment to finding and appraising information; free, high-quality evidence-based information is in much lower supply and concentration on the Internet than in the specialized resources mentioned above. The reason is simple: it is much easier and cheaper to produce low-quality, rather than high-quality, information. Nevertheless, there are many free sources of reliable information on the web, beginning with PubMed.

4. Is it time to change how you seek best evidence?

Compare the 4S approach with how you usually seek evidence-based information. Is it time to revise your tactics? If, for example, it surprises you that MEDLINE is low on the 4S list of resources for finding current best evidence, then this communication will have served a purpose. Resources for finding evidence have evolved in the past few years, and searches can be a lot quicker and more satisfying for answering clinical questions if the features of your quest match those of one of the evolved services. This is no knock against MEDLINE, which continues to serve as a premier access route to the studies and reviews that form the foundation for all the other more specialized databases reviewed above. But big rewards can be gained from becoming familiar with these new resources and using them whenever the right clinical question presents itself.

Another way to think of organizing your information needs is "prompt, pull, push". "Prompt" corresponds to the highest "S" level—"systems". When you interact with an electronic patient record or an evidence-based diagnostic or pharmacy service, it ought to prompt you if a feature of your patient corresponds to an evidence-based care guideline that you haven't already incorporated into their care plan. As indicated above, such systems are not widely available at present, although this is beginning to change. "Pull" corresponds to the three lower levels of the 4S approach: you go hunting to "pull" the evidence you need from available resources. "Push" refers to having evidence sent to you; controlling this is the subject of the next section.

HOW TO DEAL WITH THE EVIDENCE THAT FINDS YOU: KEEPING UP TO DATE EFFICIENTLY

1. Cancel your full-text journal subscriptions

Trying to keep up-to-date in your clinical practice by reading full-text journals is a truly hopeless task. From an evidence-based perspective, for a broad-based discipline such as general practice, the number of articles you need to read to find one article that meets basic criteria for quality and relevance ranges from 86 to 107 for the top five full-text general journals.[8] At, say, 2 minutes per article, that's about 3 hours to find one article ready for clinical action; and then the article may cover old ground or provide "me-too" evidence of yet-another statin, or not be useful to you because of the way you have specialized the scope of your practice. You should trade in your (traditional) journal subscriptions. It will save you time but won't necessarily save you money, because you will need to invest in better resources for keeping current (see below).

2. Invest in evidence-based journals and online services

A growing number of periodicals summarize the best evidence in traditional journals, making their selections according to explicit criteria for merit, providing structured abstracts of the best studies and expert commentaries about the context of the studies and the clinical applicability of their findings. These synoptic journals include *ACP Journal Club, Evidence Based Medicine, Evidence Based Mental Health, Evidence Based Nursing, Evidence Based Health Care Policy and Practice, Evidence Based Cardiovascular Medicine*, and a number of others. Synoptic journals do what traditional journals wish they could do in selecting the best studies, finding the best articles from all relevant journals and summarizing them in one place. Traditional journals can't do this because they can only publish from among the articles that authors choose to send them.

If you find articles on a topic of high interest to you, and these appear in a journal to which you or your institution subscribes, then you can often invoke a number of ancillary services. For example, say you were interested in the EBM Online (http://ebm.bmjjournals.com/) article, "Review: continuing treatment with antidepressants reduces the rate of relapse or recurrence of depressive symptoms regardless of duration of treatment before or after randomization". This synopsis is linked to the full-text article in *The Lancet*, so you can read the full review. You can also "click" (1) to be alerted when new articles cite this review, (2) to be connected to similar synopses in EBM Online or to similar articles in the publisher's other journals, (3) to e-mail the item to a friend or colleague, or (4) to download the synopsis to citation manager software. The synopsis is also linked to the PubMed abstract of the original article and this leads to PubMed's various features, such as "Related Articles" and "Links" to other services.

For the most part, these evidence-based synopsis journals are targeted for generalists. If you are a subspecialist, you may have to build your own current awareness service. This is easily possible through having the title pages of journals of relevance to your practice sent to you for free from such services as Cubby in MEDLINE (http://www.ncbi.nlm. nih.gov/entrez/cubby.fcgi?call=QueryExt.Quer.last. Show & call=Query Ext.CubbyQuery.Show-All), or sent to you for a price from *Current Contents*. Further, subspecialty journal clubs are sprouting on the web, such as PedsCCM *Evidence Based Journal Club* (http://pedsccm.wustl. edu/EBJournal_club. html), *Family Practice Journal Club* (POEMS) (http://www. infopoems.com/), and *Critical Care* (http://ahsn.lhsc.on.ca). It is difficult to keep track of all the new services. The ones we know about are listed on the CD and will be kept up to date on our book's website (http://www.cebm,utoronto.ca). SCHARR provides excellent links to many more evidence-based services (www.shef.ac.uk/uni/academic/R-Z/ scharr/ir/netting.html).

WALKING THE WALK
Searching for evidence to solve patient problems

As in swimming and bicycle riding, the use of evidence-based information resources is best learned by examples and practice, not by reading. Commit yourself to paper on three matters for each of the problems below before you move on to the rest of the chapter:

1. The key question to seek an answer for (using the guidelines from Ch. 1).

2. The best answer to the clinical problem that you currently have stored in your brain (being as quantitative as possible).

3. The evidence resources (both traditional and avant garde) that you would consult to find best current answers.

CLINICAL SCENARIO

Mrs Smothers, an accountant, is a moderately obese, 56-year-old white woman with type 2 diabetes, first diagnosed 3 years ago. She visits you in a somewhat agitated state. She missed her previous appointment ("tax time"), and has not been at the clinic for over a year. Her 55-year-old sister also had diabetes and recently died of a heart attack. Mrs Smothers found some information on the Internet that will allow her to calculate her own risk of heart attack, but she lacks some of the information needed to do the calculation, including her cholesterol and recent hemoglobin A_{1c}. She wants your help in completing the calculation and your advice about reducing her risk.

She is currently trying to quit her smoking habit of 25 years. She is on a prescribed regimen of a calorie-restricted diet (with no weight loss in the past year), exercise (she states about 20 minutes of walking once or twice a week, hampered by her osteoarthritis), and metformin 2500 mg/day (sometimes missed, especially when she skips meals). Mr Smothers accompanies Mrs Smothers on this visit and interjects that she is also taking vitamin E and beta-carotene to lower her risk for heart disease, based on a health advisory that Mr Smothers read on the

---

Internet. The occasional fasting blood sugars she has taken have been between 7 and 14 mmol/L (126–252 mg/dL). She hasn't had an eye examination in over a year and didn't get a `flu shot. She has no other physical complaints at present, but admits to being depressed since her sister's death. She specifically denies symptoms of chest pain, stroke, or claudication.

On examination, Mrs Smothers is 98 kg in weight and 172 cm in height. Her blood pressure is 148/86 mmHg in the left arm with a large adult cuff, repeated. The rest of her examination is unremarkable, including her optic fundi, cardiovascular system, chest, abdomen, skin, feet, and sensation.

You ask her what risk calculator she found and she shows you the web page that she printed. You tell her that you will check out the web page and enthusiastically endorse tightening up her regimen to bring her into the "green zone" for blood sugar, blood pressure, and cholesterol control. She is not keen to consume additional prescription medication, preferring "natural remedies", but states that she is open to discussion, especially in view of her sister's death. She wants to know her risk of heart attack and just how much benefit she can expect from any additional medication you might propose for her. You tell her that you will be pleased to help her get the answers to her questions, but will need to update her lab tests and have her return in 2 weeks. She is not very pleased about having to wait, but accepts your explanation. Heeding a recent dictum from your clinic manager, you order a "lean and mean" minimalist set of lab tests: hemoglobin A_{1c}, lipid profile, creatinine, urinary microalbumin:creatinine ratio, and ECG (electrocardiogram).

Write down the key questions that identify the evidence needed to give Mrs Smothers clear answers about risks from her condition and benefits from its treatments. Then indicate your best answers before searching (stick your neck out!), and select evidence resources that you feel will provide current best evidence to support answers suited to this patient.

Question:

Your best answer

Initial evidence source

At this point, you should have written down the key question, your current answer, and the evidence resources that you feel are best suited to answer these questions. Now would be a good time to try your hand at finding the answers by the routes you've selected, keeping track of how much time, ease/aggravation and money your searches cost and how satisfied you are in the end. Put yourself under some time pressure: summarize the best evidence you can find in 30 minutes or less for each question. (You may be thinking about skipping this exercise, hoping that the rest of this chapter will teach you how to do it effortlessly. But there is wisdom in the maxim "no pain, no gain". Invest at least 30 minutes of your time on at least one of the questions before you press on.)

What follows is based on the general approach, described at the beginning of this chapter, to identifying and using key evidence-based resources. It is important to note that there may be more than one good route (not to mention a myriad of bad routes), and that, as this book ages, better routes will assuredly be built. Indeed, many improved resources have become available since publication of the second edition of this book in 2000, and resources such as EBMR, *Clinical Evidence*, and the Cochrane Library, have greatly matured. Thus, one of the foundations of providing efficient, evidence-based health care is keeping tabs on the availability, scope and quality of new resources that are directly pertinent to our own professional practice.

If you have tried to search for evidence on these problems, compare what you did and what you found with our methods. If you haven't tried to search yet, we issue you a challenge: see if you can find a better answer than we did (we searched in late 2003, but we won't begrudge you a better answer that you found after this time). Updates on effective searching strategies, including especially those that our readers create (if you find a better answer, e-mail your

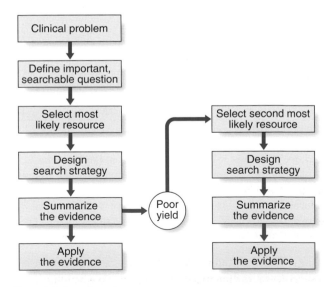

Figure 2.2 General search strategy.

strategy to us through our website), will appear (with attribution) on this book's website (www.cebm.utoronto.ca).

Carrying out the searching steps

Basic steps for acquiring the evidence to support a clinical decision are shown in Figure 2.2. We've supplied the clinical problem, and have asked you to take the first step, defining the questions to be answered, following the lead in Chapter 1. Have a go at it if you haven't done so already. Here's our try for the example above.

Problem
Type 2 diabetes and related cardiovascular risk.

Step 1. Asking answerable questions

Investigations have shown that Mrs Smothers has an A_{1c} of 8.9%, microproteinuria and hyperlipidemia, with total cholesterol 6.48 mmol/L, LDL 3.4 mmol/L, HDL 0.9 mmol/L, and triglycerides 3.9 mmol/L. With this additional information, we pose the question: In a 56-year-old woman with type 2 diabetes mellitus, microproteinuria, elevated blood pressure, and dyslipidemia, what is the evidence concerning increased risk for cardiovascular complications compared with people with diabetes without these risk factors (and does the risk calculator that Mrs Smothers found provide an evidence-based estimate of risk that fits her circumstances)? In such a patient, does "tight" control of glucose, blood pressure, cholesterol, and proteinuria reduce subsequent morbidity and mortality?

Step 2A. Selecting an evidence resource

Step 2A is to decide where to search. The example in this chapter is drawn from the practice of internal medicine, so the focus will be on the best and quickest evidence-based information sources for this clinical discipline, including general and specialized bibliographic databases, in both print and electronic form.

For the most part, electronic media with periodic updates (especially on the Internet, with CD valuable when the Internet is not readily accessible) are rendering paper sources obsolete for looking up evidence. Electronic media are generally much more accessible, much more thoroughly indexed, and, most importantly, have the potential to be much more up-to-date than paper-based resources. Moreover, hypertext and the Internet permit unlimited linkages to related and supplementary information. Thus, a good computer (whether ours or someone else's) with an Internet link (or at least a CD-ROM drive), and a working knowledge of the evidence resources that have been developed for our own clinical discipline, can make an important difference to whether we will be successful in becoming evidence-based practitioners.

How to deal with the evidence that finds you

The first piece of information to consider in this case falls into the general category of "evidence that finds you"; as in our case for example, patients frequently find information that they want you to comment on, so you need an efficient approach to evaluating the pedigree and evidence base for claims they encounter on the Internet or other media. This patient brought along a web page (http://www.betterdiabetescare.org/TOOLBOXrisk.htm) that she had found through Google, so it was easy to examine this source. This website has impeccable credentials, with material prepared by the National Diabetes Education Program with sponsorship from the US National Institutes of Health, the National Institute of Diabetes and Digestive and Kidney Diseases, and Centers for Disease Control, and without commercial advertising. This is not to say that the information on the website is necessarily either accurate or up-to-date, but it is more likely to be so than websites that lack these features. You breathe a sigh of relief for such an easy search.

Two risk calculators for cardiovascular disease are offered on the website, one from Framingham, which can be done with a pencil and paper (http://www.nhlbi.nih.gov/about/framingham/riskwom.pdf), the other from the UK (http://www.dtu.ox.ac.uk/index.html?maindoc=/riskengine/). Both are supported by published studies.

Because the UK calculator was specifically developed among patients with diabetes and is more recent, you retrieve the relevant study cited.[9] Details in this report indicate that the patients were an "inception cohort" of 4540 newly diagnosed patients with type 2 diabetes mellitus, followed for a median of over 10 years, with close monitoring for cardiovascular and other complications, and with very few patients being lost to follow-up or having missing data. As you will learn in Chapter 4, these features mean that the study meets critical appraisal criteria for the validity of prognostic studies. You decide to download the risk calculator to your computer and fire it up. You plug in the lab results for Mrs Smothers and the display is as shown in Figure 2.3.

Thus, Mrs Smothers has a substantial absolute risk of experiencing the onset of coronary heart disease during the coming decade, namely 27.3%. Her risk of stroke is also elevated. You note that the website offers a Palm version and download that for future use in your clinic. Both versions will allow you to "play" with the figures, monitoring your patient's status over time as test results change, and estimating the effect of interventions that alter the lab results.

For consistency, you check the Framingham risk calculator. This is based on the famous Framingham Study in the USA and is derived from a cohort of 5345 people initially free of coronary heart disease (CHD), who were followed beginning in 1971–74.[10] Only about 3% of Framingham participants had diabetes at the beginning of observation, and it could have been present for any length of time before entering the study. Thus, this study would not meet the validity criteria for studying the prognosis of diabetes. It does, however, meet basic criteria for appraising the validity of studies of etiology/harm (covered in Ch. 6). Thus, we are justified in looking at its prediction of risk for patients such as ours. We select the chart for predicting CHD risk for women, based on LDL-cholesterol. Given her characteristics and lab values, the risk score for Mrs Smothers would be 19, associated with a 10-year CHD risk of >32%, about three times the average risk for her age group. It is reassuring (statistically, if not clinically!) that this estimate is at the upper limit of the 95% confidence interval of the risk

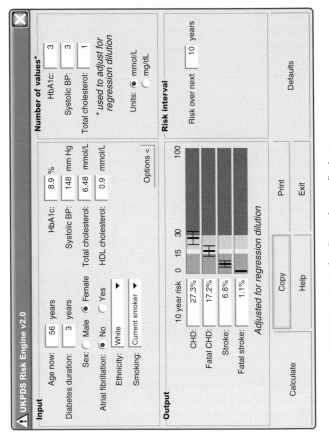

Figure 2.3 UKPDS Risk Engine estimate of cardiovascular complications.

estimate we obtained from the UKPDS risk tool. The lower estimated UKPDS risk is consistent with patients in UKPDS being earlier in the course of their diabetes, and with better management of diabetes and cardiovascular risk factors in UKPDS (conducted in the 1990s) than Framingham (which followed patients during the 1970s and 1980s).

Where to find the best evidence

For a woman of her age, Mrs Smothers certainly has a high risk of experiencing a CHD event or stroke in the coming years. It might seem that we already have the evidence to proceed—indeed, an imperative to intervene. But she has asked us to provide evidence that our interventions will help (compared with, say, the vitamin E and beta-carotene her husband told us about), and rightly so. The intervention question we posed was: In patients like her, does "tight" control of glucose, blood pressure, cholesterol, and proteinuria reduce subsequent morbidity and mortality?

Using the 4S approach, we begin with Ovid, the "4S supermarket", and head for *Clinical Evidence*, a *system* that integrates current best evidence for specified clinical questions. Described earlier in this chapter, Ovid provides several evidence-based resources and databases, and is currently one of the most comprehensive evidence-based "aggregator" services available. As a result, it will most often be a premier resource for one-stop shopping. That will not necessarily make it the best resource for a given question, but it is the right place to start if you have access to Ovid and you don't know exactly what the best source is.

Step 2B. Executing the search strategy

Using our library's Ovid access from home (by proxy service; if you don't already have this set up on your computer, your library's home page likely tells you how to do this), with a cable modem, we look up *Clinical Evidence*, browse the table of contents to Endocrine Disorders, and see five subtopics, two of which are "Cardiovascular disease in diabetes" and "Glycemic control in diabetes". The first of these topics links to a

Table 2.2 Summary of evidence for the management of diabetes and conditions

Study	Interventions	Study type	Duration (years)	Outcome	Events/sample size (%) Intervention	Events/sample size (%) Control	NNT	95% CI for NNT
Antihypertensive medication								
UKPDS	"Tight" target BP (≤150/≤85) with captopril or atenolol vs. "less-tight" target (≤180/≤105)	RCT	8.4	AMI (fatal or non-fatal) stroke	107/758 (14%) 38/758 (5.0%)	83/390 (21%) 34/390 (8.7%)	14 27	9 to 35 18 to 116
				Peripheral vascular events	8/758 (1.1%)	8/390 (2.1%)	ND	ND
HOT	Felodipine and ACE inhibitor, or beta-blocker, with three distinct target BPs	RCT	3.8	AMI (fatal or non-fatal), stroke (fatal or non-fatal), or other cardiovascular death	22/499 (4.4%) Target diastolic BP 80 mmHg	45/501 (9.0%) Target diastolic BP 90 mmHg	22	16 to 57
FACET	Fosinopril vs. amiodipine	RCT	2.9	AMI, stroke, or admission to hospital for angina	14/189 (7.4%) Fosinopril	27/191 (14%) Amiodipine	15	10 to 199
ABCD	Enalapril vs. nisoldipine	RCT	5	AMI (fatal or non-fatal) MI, CHF, or sudden cardiac death	5/235 (2.1%) Enalapril	25/235 (11%) Nisoldipine	12	10 to 19

Syst-Eur	Nitrendipine; enalapril± hydrochlorothiazide (20 mmHg BP lowering) vs. placebo	RCT	2	MI, CHF, or sudden cardiac death	13/252 (5%)	31/240 (13%)	13	10 to 31
Lipid-regulating agents								
AFCAPS/ ToxCAPS	Lovastatin	RCT	5	MI, unstable angina, or sudden cardiac death	4/84 (4.8%)	6/71 (8.5%)	27	NS
SENDCAP	Bezafibrate	RCT	3	MI, or new ischemic changes on ECG	5/64 (7.8%)	16/64 (25%)	6	5 to 20
Helsinki	Gemfibrozil	RCT	5	MI or cardiac death	2/59 (3.4%)	8/76 (10.5%)	14	NS
HPS	Simvastatin vs. placebo	RCT	5	CHD, stroke, revascularization	133/1455 (9.1%)	197/1457 (13.5%)	23	15 to 48

Table 2.2 (cont'd)

Study	Interventions	Study type	Duration (years)	Outcome	Events/sample size (%) Intervention	Events/sample size (%) Control	NNT	95% CI for NNT
Blood glucose control								
UKPDS	Intensive treatment with insulin and/or sulfonylurea vs. conventional treatment	RCT	5	MI (fatal or non-fatal)	387/2729 (14.2%)	186/1138 (16.3%)	46	NS
UKPDS	Intensive treatment with metformin vs. conventional treatment	RCT	5	MI (fatal or non-fatal)	39/342 (11%)	73/411 (18%)	16	10 to 71
DCCT	Intensive insulin treatment in type 1 diabetes	RCT	6.5	Major macrovascular events	23/711 (3.2%)	40/730 (5.5%)	45	28 to 728
Aspirin								
Physicians' Health Study	Aspirin	RCT	5	MI (fatal or non-fatal)	11/275 (4.0%)	26/258 (10%)	16	12 to 47
ETDRS (mixed primary and secondary prevention)	Aspirin	RCT	5	MI (fatal or non-fatal)	289/1856 (15.6%)	336/1855 (18.1%)	39	21 to 716

Reproduced from *Clinical Evidence*, with permission of the BMJ Publishing Group.

summary of interventions organized in three categories ("beneficial," "likely to be beneficial", and "unknown effectiveness"), followed by key messages. We click on the first beneficial treatment link, "antihypertensive treatment", which leads us to an evidence summary table: "Primary prevention of cardiovascular events in people with diabetes: evidence from systematic reviews and randomized trials". This section summarizes several recent trials with quantitative results (including "number needed to treat", NNT; see Appendix 2 for a definition if you don't already know what this means), showing cardiovascular benefits from lowering blood pressure, lipids, and blood sugar as well as from prescribing aspirin. You bookmark and print the table for reference when you have completed your search (see Table 2.2; accessed in December 2003 and likely changed now).

Three minutes and the search is essentially done, except for one detail: you noticed as you were entering the diabetes cardiovascular section in *Clinical Evidence* that the literature search for this section was done in April 2002, whereas the search we've just completed above was in December 2003. It is good news that the date of last search is posted within each section in *Clinical Evidence*, but it is not so good news that this section has not been revised in so long. While the table you retrieved appears to have more than enough evidence to proceed, it may be worthwhile to check another source. Again, we'll look for a system: *UpToDate*. This is not part of Ovid's collection. You may be affiliated with an institution that subscribes to it, as ours does; otherwise you will need to acquire a subscription yourself.*

A search in *UpToDate* for "diabetes" retrieves a number of titles, and we select "Diabetes mellitus, type 2". This search retrieves more than a page of subtopics so we click the "Narrow the search results" button beside the search window and select "Treatment", and then select "Overview of therapy in type 2 diabetes mellitus". This section

---

* Note, that we could have clicked on EBMR and *Clinical Evidence* on the Ovid main page and searched these resources simultaneously. We would find both the *Clinical Evidence* entry and the relevant abstract and commentary from *ACP Journal Club* with just one search.

summarizes treatments, including aspirin, and medications for lowering blood sugar, blood pressure, cholesterol and triglycerides, and screening for complications such as retinopathy. Further, the chapter summarizes the benefits of "Multifactorial risk factor reduction", citing a trial published in 2003 by Gaede et al,[11] showing the benefits for patients of therapy that is directed to reducing all risk factors to low levels.

The Gaede trial looks like just the thing to focus the discussion for Mrs Smothers. The abstract for this study is provided in *UpToDate*, along with its PubMed ID. We "copy" the PubMed ID and "paste" it in the search box for PubMed. The search instantly retrieves the article's abstract along with links to the full-text article describing the *study* and to its *synopsis* in *ACP Journal Club*.

For the sake of comparison, we looked at some other sources. The Gaede study is summarized in *ACP Journal Club*. *ACP Medicine*, accessed via the web, had a detailed chapter on diabetes, written by one of the leading experts in the field, but the date of preparation for this chapter was 2001, 2 years before the Gaede study was published. *Harrison's Principles of Internal of Medicine*, accessed via Harrison's Online, displayed a copyright claim for the period 2001–2003, but the most recent reference in the diabetes section (Ch. 33) was dated 2000. This text also does not link assertions and recommendations in the text to specific citations of evidence. Thus, the take-home message is that we need to know how and when a text, CD, or Internet site was constructed to ensure that important new advances are being incorporated quickly. Failing that, the resource should at least provide references linked directly to key content so we can discern the date of publication of the evidence that is cited. We could have looked at a traditional, printed textbook as well but this is usually a waste of time unless it's been recently released. Indeed, for printed books, months pass between when chapters are written and when the print version is released and therefore they can be out-of-date on the date of publication!

Step 2C. Examining the evidence

Discounting the side-trip to more traditional textbooks, we've quickly assembled the *system*, *synopsis*, and *study* level information needed to inform an evidence-based decision for Mrs Smothers. The Gaede study is summarized in *ACP Journal Club*, so it has already passed muster for scientific merit and we can skip this critical appraisal step unless we want to look for details that don't appear in the *ACP Journal Club* abstract. The study investigated the benefits of intensive management of type 2 diabetes in a diabetes clinic compared with conventional care by family practitioners with open access to consultation. The findings from this study appear in Tables 2.3 and 2.4.

The study showed an improvement in the process of care for the treatment goals for hemoglobin A_{1c}, cholesterol, triglycerides, and systolic blood pressure (Table 2.3). More importantly, it showed significant reductions in adverse

Table 2.3 Percentage of patients with type 2 diabetes meeting treatment goals, 8 years into care

	Conventional care (%)	Intensive care (%)
Hemoglobin A_{1c} <6.5%	3	16
Total cholesterol <4.5 L	20	72
Triglycerides <1.7 mmol/L	45	58
Systolic blood pressure <130 mmHg	18	45

Table 2.4 RCT of intensive vs. conventional treatment for patients with type 2 diabetes and persistent proteinuria

	Relative risk reduction (%)	95% CI
Cardiovascular system outcomes	53	27 to 76
Diabetic nephropathy	61	13 to 83
Retinopathy	58	14 to 79
Autonomic neuropathy	63	21 to 82

cardiovascular outcomes, diabetic nephropathy, retinopathy, and neuropathy (Table 2.4). The absolute risk reduction in cardiovascular events was 20% (24% in the intervention group vs. 44% in the control group) over the 8-year average follow-up in the trial, giving an NNT of five patients to prevent one additional cardiovascular event. (The details of how these calculations are done are covered in Chapter 5. Therapy and the basic definitions and calculations are given in Appendix 2.)

Practice makes perfect

For further practice in finding the best evidence, you might want to tackle the question of whether vitamin E and beta-carotene are Mrs Smothers' friends, foes, or just more fees for her.

Step 1. Asking an answerable question

> In high cardiovascular risk smokers, do vitamin E and beta-carotene prevent clinical events or death, compared with not taking these chemicals?

Step 2A. Selecting an evidence resource + Step 2B. Executing the search strategy + Step 2C. Examining the evidence

A quick search (30 seconds) of *ACP Journal Club* (www.acpjc.org) for beta-carotene retrieved 12 items, including a recent systematic review of large trials of antioxidant vitamins, vitamin E or beta-carotene, for the primary or secondary prevention of mortality or cardiovascular disease.[12] All-cause mortality and cardiovascular deaths were increased in the people taking beta-carotene compared with control interventions (usually placebo); vitamin E conferred no benefit.

It hardly seems necessary to look further, but *Clinical Evidence* and *UpToDate* both review "antioxidant vitamins" with the same conclusions. (Note that, using our 4S approach, we could have searched *Clinical Evidence* first and followed it with our synopsis search.) With all this evidence showing no benefit of antioxidants, you begin to wonder what the hype about them is about . . . and why beta-carotene is still available over-the-counter, alone, and as a common constituent of multivitamins. Should you post a warning on the wall of your office?

Harrison's Principles of Internal Medicine and *ACP Medicine* also cited two trials describing adverse effects from beta-carotene in lung cancer prevention, but neither provided findings for cardiovascular disease. A Cochrane Library search on beta-carotene retrieved no reviews in CDSR, two reviews in DARE, and many trial and review references in the Cochrane Central Register of Controlled Trials.

Just for practice, try your hand with PubMed (http://www.ncbi.nlm.nih.gov/PubMed/) and PubMed Clinical Queries (http://www.ncbi.nlm.nih.gov/entrez/query/static/clinical.html). A search on beta-carotene or vitamin E using PubMed (in December 2003) retrieves 27 168 references! Although most of them have something to do with the general topic, we gave up when the first 20 citations did not appear to address our question directly. Switching to PubMed's Clinical Queries, selecting the Systematic Reviews option and using the same search terms, the review summarized in *ACP Journal Club* is found ninth in the list of 152 citations, following eight citations that appear to be less pertinent. Adding "mortality and cardiovascular" to the search strategy (i.e. "beta-carotene and vitamin E and mortality and cardiovascular") reduces the yield to 61 citations of which the systematic review is fourth. So many roads lead to a current systematic review of the evidence, but some roads are a lot shorter and smoother than others.

Applying the evidence

Evidence can bring you a long way towards helping Mrs Smothers with her problems, including gaining an accurate prognosis, determining current best methods for reducing her risks for adverse cardiovascular and diabetes outcomes, and providing her with information concerning non-prescribed treatments she is taking. However, it is important to observe that "evidence does not make decisions". Other key components are her clinical circumstances and her wishes.[2]

It is important to note that she has a number of medical problems: obesity, poorly controlled diabetes, hypertension, dyslipidemia, and she smokes. Dealing with all these problems simultaneously is unlikely to occur because of the heavy behavioral demands of the complex regimen that would be required to treat them all successfully. You will need to negotiate priorities carefully with the patient to find the best match between the evidence and her wishes, then incorporate current best evidence concerning interventions to help her follow the treatments that she has agreed to accept.[13] Thus, the evidence you have accumulated in this chapter will get you only part of the way towards the decisions that Mrs Smothers and you will need to make, but at least your decisions will be informed by the best available evidence concerning her risks and the interventions that will reduce or, in the case of beta-carotene, increase them. We'll discuss the application of evidence about therapy in further detail in Chapter 5.

There are many other ways of tracking down relevant evidence with which to answer our clinical questions and we've provided only a couple of approaches here. Moreover, our discussion has focused primarily on questions of therapy and prognosis. If we have a different type of clinical question, we'd need to match our question to relevant resources and modify our search strategy accordingly. For example, if our question is one of diagnosis, we wouldn't start with *Clinical Evidence* since it doesn't include diagnostic evidence. Similarly, the Cochrane Library does not include diagnostic reviews as of this date, although they will be forthcoming. We've provided some examples of potential search cascades for these types of searches on the accompanying CD.

REFERENCES

1 Quote in Pickering GW. BMJ 1956; 2: 113–16.

2 Haynes RB, Devereaux PJ, Guyatt GH. Clinical expertise in the era of evidence-based medicine and patient choice [editorial]. ACP J Club 2002; 136: A11–13.

3 Hunt DL, Haynes RB, Hanna SE, Smith K. Effects of computer-based clinical decision support systems on physician performance and patient outcomes: a systematic review. JAMA 1998; 280: 1339–46.

4 UpToDate. UpToDate in Medicine. Wellesley, MA: BDR Inc.

5 Dale DC, ed. WebMD Scientific American Medicine. New York: Scientific American Medicine (Internet, serial CD-ROM, print).

6 Braunwald E, Fauci AS, Isselbacher KJ, Kasper DL, Hauser SL, Longo DL, et al, eds. Harrison's Principles of Internal Medicine, 15th edn. Philadelphia: McGraw-Hill, 2001.

7 Review: Low-molecular-weight heparin is effective and safe in the acute coronary syndromes [abstract]. ACP J Club 2003; 139: 58. Abstract for Wong GC, Giugliano RP, Antman EM. Use of low-molecular-weight heparins in the management of acute coronary artery syndromes and percutaneous coronary intervention. JAMA 2003; 289: 331–42 (http://www.acpjc.org/Content/139/3/issue/ACPJC-2003-139-3-058.htm).

8 McKibbon KA, Wilczynski NL, Haynes RB. What do evidence-based secondary journals tell us about the clinical meat in primary health care journals? BMC Med (to be submitted).

9 Stevens RJ, Kothari V, Adler AI, Stratton IM, and United Kingdom Prospective Diabetes Study (UKPDS) Group. The UKPDS risk engine: a model for the risk of coronary heart disease in type II diabetes (UKPDS 56). Clin Sci (Lond) 2001; 101: 671–9.

10 Wilson PWF, D'Agostino RB, Levy D, Balanger AM, Silbershatz H, Kannell WB. Prediction of coronary heart disease using risk factor categories. Circulation 1998; 97: 1837–47.

11 Gaede P, Vedel P, Larsen N, Jensen GV, Parving HH, Pedersen O. Multifactorial intervention and cardiovascular disease in patients with type 2 diabetes. N Engl J Med 2003; 348: 383–93.

12 Review: Prophylactic use of beta-carotene may increase the risk for all-cause mortality and cardiovascular death [abstract]. ACP J Club 2004; 140. Vivekananthan DP, Penn MS, Sapp SK, Hsu A, Topol EJ. Use of antioxidant vitamins for the prevention of cardiovascular disease: meta-analysis of randomised trials. Lancet 2003; 361: 2017–23.

13 Review: Evidence on the effectiveness of interventions to assist patient adherence to prescribed medications is limited [abstract]. ACP J Club 2002; 139: 19. McDonald HP, Garg AX, Haynes RB. Interventions to enhance patient adherence to medication prescriptions: scientific review. JAMA 2002; 288: 2868–79.

Diagnosis and screening

Dx

In this chapter we will help you answer three questions about diagnostic tests:

1. Is this evidence about the accuracy of a diagnostic test valid?

2. Does this (valid) evidence show that this test can accurately distinguish patients who do and do not have a specific disorder?

3. How can I apply this valid, accurate diagnostic test to a specific patient?

3

After retrieving evidence about a test's accuracy, questions 1 and 2 suggest we need to decide if it's valid and important before we can apply the evidence to our individual patients. As with therapy, the order in which we consider validity and importance is not crucial, and depends on individual preference, but both should be done before applying the study results. Because the screening and early diagnosis of symptomless individuals have some similarities with, but also some crucial differences from, the diagnosis of sick ones, we'll close with a special section devoted to these acts at the interface of clinical medicine and public health.

Figure 3.1 shows the post-test probabilities after positive (upper curve) and negative (lower curve) test results for the range of possible pre-test probabilities of disease. The first question, on validity, asks if we can believe the information in the graph. The second question, on importance, asks if the results show clinically worthwhile shifts in uncertainty (the further apart the post-test curves, the larger this shift). The third question means we need to understand how the test results might change our diagnostic uncertainty on application, not only for the patients in the study but, more importantly, for a particular patient.

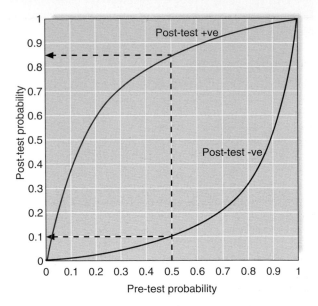

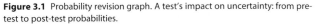

Figure 3.1 Probability revision graph. A test's impact on uncertainty: from pre-test to post-test probabilities.

To illustrate our discussion, we'll consider the following patient.

CLINICAL SCENARIO

Suppose that we're working up a patient with anemia and think that the probability that she has iron-deficiency anemia is 50% (i.e. the odds are about 50:50 that the anemia is due to iron deficiency). When we present the patient to our boss, we ask for an educational prescription to determine the usefulness of performing a serum ferritin on our patient as a means of detecting iron-deficiency anemia. By the time we've tracked down and studied the external evidence, our patient's serum ferritin comes back at 60 mmol/L. How should we put all this together?

Before looking at the scenario and our three questions, we should take a short detour through the land of "abnormality" so that what we might understand what could be meant by a normal or an abnormal ferritin.

WHAT IS (AB)NORMAL?

Most test reports will wind up calling some results "normal" and others "abnormal". There are at least six definitions of "normal" in common use (listed in Table 3.1). This chapter will focus on definition 5 ("diagnostic" normal), because we think that the first four definitions have important flaws. The first two (the gaussian and percentile definitions) focus just on the diagnostic test results in either a normal (the left-hand cluster in Figure 3.2) or an undifferentiated group of people (an unknown mix of the left and right clusters in Figure 3.2), with no reference standard. They define the "normal range" on the basis of statistical properties (standard deviations or percentiles). They not only imply that all "abnormalities" occur at the same frequency, but suggest that, if we perform more and more diagnostic tests on our patient, we are increasingly likely to find something "abnormal", thus leading to all sorts of inappropriate further testing.

The third definition of "normal" (culturally desirable) represents the sorts of value judgment seen in fashion

---

Table 3.1 Six definitions of normal

1. **Gaussian**: the mean±2 standard deviations; this assumes a normal distribution for all tests and results in all "abnormalities" having the same frequency.

2. **Percentile**: within the range, say of 5–95%; has the same basic defect as the gaussian definition.

3. **Culturally desirable**: when "normal" is that which is preferred by society, the role of medicine gets confused.

4. **Risk factor**: carrying no additional risk of disease; nicely labels the outliers, but does changing a risk factor necessarily change risk?

5. **Diagnostic**: range of results beyond which target disorders become highly probable; the focus of this discussion.

6. **Therapeutic**: range of results beyond which treatment does more good than harm; means we have to keep up with advances in therapy!

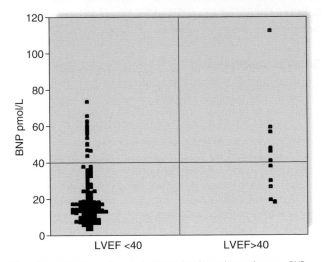

Figure 3.2 Distribution of results in diseased and non-diseased groups. BNP, brain natriuretic peptide; LVEF, left ventricular ejection fraction. (Adapted with permission from Smith H, Pickering RM, Struthers A, et al. BMJ 2000; 320: 906–8.)

advertisements, and at the fringes of the "lifestyle" movement where medicine becomes confused with morality. The fourth (risk factor) definition has the drawback that it "labels" or stigmatizes some patients regardless of whether we can intervene to lower their risk—a big problem with neonatal genetic testing and other screening maneuvers, as you'll learn in the concluding section of this chapter. The fifth (diagnostic) definition is the one that we will focus on here, and we will show you how to work with it in the next bit of this chapter. The final (therapeutic) definition (does treating at and beyond this level do more good than harm?) is in part an outgrowth of the fourth (risk factor) definition, but has the great clinical advantage that it changes with our knowledge of efficacy. Thus, the definition of normal blood pressure has changed radically over the past few decades as we have learned that treatment of progressively less pronounced elevations of blood pressure does more good than harm.

IS THIS EVIDENCE ABOUT THE ACCURACY OF A DIAGNOSTIC TEST VALID?

Having found a possibly useful article about a diagnostic test, how can we quickly critically appraise it for its proximity to the truth? The questions listed in Table 3.2 are for individual reports, but we can also apply them to the interpretation of a systematic review (overview) of several different studies of the same diagnostic test for the same target disorder.*

Table 3.2 Is this evidence about a diagnostic test valid?

1. **Measurement**: was the reference ("gold") standard measured independently, i.e. blind to our target test?

2. **Representative**: was the diagnostic test evaluated in an appropriate spectrum of patients (like those in whom we would use it in practice)?

3. **Ascertainment**: was the reference standard ascertained regardless of the diagnostic test result?

(Fourth question to be considered for clusters of tests of clinical prediction rules: was the cluster of tests validated in a second, independent group of patients?)

---

1. Measurement: Was there an independent, blind comparison with a reference ("gold") standard?†

The patients in the study should have undergone both the diagnostic test in question (say, an item of the history or physical examination, a blood test, etc.) and the reference (or

---

* As we'll stress throughout this book, systematic reviews provide us with the most valid and useful external evidence on just about any clinical question we can pose. They are still pretty rare for diagnostic tests and for this reason we'll describe them in their usual, therapeutic habitat, in Chapter 5. When applying Table 5.9 to diagnostic tests, simply substitute "diagnostic test" for "treatment" as you read.

† Note: to approximate the sequence of steps in the critical appraisal of therapy articles, we could consider the appraisal questions using the order representativeness, ascertainment, and measurement. You'll notice that the first letters of these words produce the acronym "RAM", which some learners might find useful for remembering the appraisal questions. Alternatively, when considering the validity of reports of diagnostic test accuracy, others might find it easier to consider the most crucial question first: Was there a comparison with an appropriate reference standard? If an appropriate reference standard was not used, we can toss the article without reading further, thereby becoming more efficient knowledge managers.

"gold") standard (an autopsy or biopsy or other confirmatory "proof" that they do or do not have the target disorder). Sometimes investigators have a difficult time coming up with clear-cut reference standards (e.g. for psychiatric disorders), and we'll want to give careful consideration to their arguments justifying the selection of their reference standard. Moreover, we caution you against the uncritical acceptance of reference standards, even when they are based on "expert" interpretations of biopsies; for example, in an *Evidence Based Medicine* note, Kenneth Fleming[1] reported that the degree of agreement over and above chance in reading breast, skin and liver biopsies is less than 50%! The results of one test should not be known to the folk who are applying and interpreting the other. (For example, the decision to complete the biopsy should not be dependent on the result of the diagnostic test under study, and the pathologist interpreting the biopsy that comprises the reference standard for the target disorder should be "blind" to the result of the blood test that comprises the diagnostic test under study.) In this way, investigators avoid the conscious and unconscious bias that might otherwise cause the reference standard to be "over-interpreted" when the diagnostic test is positive and "under-interpreted" when it is negative.

2. Representative: Was the diagnostic test evaluated in an appropriate spectrum of patients (like those in whom we would use it in practice)?

Did the report include patients with all the common presentations of the target disorder (including those with its early manifestations), and patients with other commonly confused diagnoses? Studies that confine themselves to florid cases vs. asymptomatic volunteers (a diagnostic "case–control" study) are useful only as a first crude check of the test, because when the diagnosis is obvious to the eye we don't need any diagnostic test. The really useful articles will be set in the diagnostic dilemmas we face, and include patients with mild as well as severe symptoms, early as well as late cases of the target disorder, and among both treated and untreated individuals.

3. Ascertainment: Was the reference standard ascertained regardless of the diagnostic test result?

When patients have a negative diagnostic test result, investigators are tempted to forego the reference standard, and when the latter is invasive or risky (e.g. angiography) it may be wrong to carry it out on patients with negative test results. To overcome this, many investigators now employ a reference standard for proving that a patient does not have the target disorder; this requires that the patient doesn't suffer any adverse health outcome during a long follow-up despite the absence of any definitive treatment (for example, convincing evidence that a patient with clinically suspected deep vein thrombosis did not have this disorder would include no ill-effects during a prolonged follow-up despite the absence of antithrombotic therapy).

If the report we're reading fails one or more of these three tests, we'll need to consider whether it has a fatal flaw that renders its conclusions invalid. If so, it's back to more searching (either now or later; if we've already used up our time for this week, perhaps we can interest a colleague or trainee in taking this on as an "educational prescription"—see p. 26 if this term is new to you). On the other hand, if the report passes this initial scrutiny and we decide that we can believe its results, and we haven't already carried out the second critical appraisal step of deciding whether these results are important, then we can proceed to the next section.

DOES THIS VALID EVIDENCE DEMONSTRATE AN IMPORTANT ABILITY OF THIS TEST TO ACCURATELY DISTINGUISH PATIENTS WHO DO AND DON'T HAVE A SPECIFIC DISORDER?

Sensitivity, specificity, and likelihood ratios

In deciding whether the evidence about a diagnostic test is important, we will focus on the accuracy of the test in distinguishing patients with and without the target disorder. We'll consider the ability of a valid test to change our minds from what we thought before the test (we'll call that the "pre-test" probability of some target disorder) to what we think afterwards (we'll call that the "post-test" probability of the target disorder). Diagnostic tests that produce big changes from pre-test to post-test probabilities are important and likely to be useful to us in our practice.

Returning to our clinical scenario, suppose further that, in filling our prescription, we find a systematic review of several studies of this diagnostic test (evaluated against the reference standard of a bone marrow stain for iron), decide that it is valid (based on the guides in Table 3.2), and find their results as shown in Table 3.3. The prevalence (or study pre-test probability) overall is 809/2579=31%. For low ferritin (<65 mmol/L), the post-test probability of iron deficiency anemia *among patients in the studies* is a/(a+b)=731/1001=73%. This study post-test probability is known as the "positive predictive value". For high ferritin (>65 mmol/L),

Table 3.3 Results of a systematic review of serum ferritin as a diagnostic test for iron deficiency anemia

| | | Target disorder (iron deficiency anemia) | | |
		Present	Absent	Totals
Diagnostic test result (serum ferritin)	Positive (<65 mmol/L)	731 a	270 b	1001 a+b
	Negative (≥65 mmol/L)	c 78	d 1500	c+d 1578
Totals		a+c 809	b+d 1770	a+b+c+d 2579

Data from: Guyatt GH, Oxman AD, Ali M, et al. J Gen Intern Med 1992; 7: 145–53.

Prevalence = (a + c)/(a + b + c + d) = 809/2579 = 31%.

Positive predictive value = a/(a + b) = 731/1001 = 73%.

Negative predictive value = d/(c + d) = 1500/1578 = 95%.

Sensitivity = a/(a + c) = 731/809 = 90%.

Specificity = d/(b + d) = 1500/1770 = 85%.

LR+ = sensitivity/(1 − specificity) = 90%/15% = 6.

LR − = (1 − sensitivity)/specificity = 10%/85% = 0.12.

Study pre-test odds=prevalence/(1 − prevalence) = 31%/69% = 0.45.

Post-test odds = pre-test odds × likelihood ratio.

Post-test probability = post-test odds/(post-test odds + 1).

the post-test probability of iron deficiency anemia *among patients in the studies* is $c/(c + d) = 78/1578 = 5\%$. This study post-test probability of 5% means that the study probability of not having iron deficiency anemia after a negative result is 95%; this is known as the "negative predictive value". So, within the study, the uncertainty regarding iron deficiency has been shifted from the initial 31% to probabilities of either 73% or 5%, which appear to be clinically important shifts.

But we thought our patient's pre-test probability of iron deficiency anemia was greater than that in the study; in fact, we estimated it to be 50%. We could do a direct adjustment of the predictive values for the patient's different pre-test probability using the following equation:

Patient post-test odds = (study post-test odds) × [(patient pre-test odds)/(study pre-test odds)]

which is analogous to the adjustment of a therapy trial's NNT (number needed to treat) for the patient's PEER (patient's expected event rate; see Ch. 5). This is fine if you have the study in hand, but generally it is easier to derive some test accuracy measures (sensitivity, specificity, and likelihood ratios) and apply these directly to the patient's individual pre-test probability. So let's look at these measures.

As you can see from Table 3.3, our patient's result (60 mmol/L) places her in the top row of the table, either in cell "a" or in cell "b". You might note from Table 3.3 that 90% of patients with iron deficiency have serum ferritin in the same range as our patient [a/(a+c)]; that property, the proportion of patients with the target disorder who have positive test results, is called "sensitivity". The sensitivity of a test is defined as the probability of a positive test given the presence of the target disorder. In diagnostic studies, we sometimes see a description of the proportion of patients who don't have the target disorder and who have negative (or normal) test results; this is called the "specificity". Returning to our patient, you might also note that only 15% of patients with other causes of their anemia have results in the same range as our patient.*

This means that our patient's result would be about six times as likely (90%/15% = 6) to be seen in someone with iron deficiency anemia as in someone without the condition; that ratio is called the "likelihood ratio" for a positive test result (LR+). The likelihood ratio for a positive test result is:

LR+= (probability of positive test in presence of target disorder)/(probability of positive test in absence of target disorder)

Since we thought ahead of time (before we had the result of the serum ferritin) that our patient's odds of iron deficiency were 50:50, that's called a "pre-test odds" of 1:1. As you can see from the formulae towards the bottom of Table 3.3, we can multiply the pre-test odds of 1 by the likelihood ratio of 6 to get the "post-test odds" of iron deficiency anemia after the test ($1 \times 6 = 6$); that's a post-test odds of 6:1 in favor of iron deficiency anemia. Since, like most clinicians, you may be more comfortable thinking in terms of probabilities than odds, this post-test odds of 6:1 converts (as you can see at the bottom of Table 3.3) to a post-test probability of 6/(6+1) = 6/7 = 86%. (To check yourself out on these calculations, try calculating the post-test probability for the same ferritin result for a patient who, like those in Table 3.3, has a pre-test odds of 0.45.† You'll know you did it right if you wind up with an answer for post-test probability that is identical to its equivalent, the positive predictive value.)

Note that we could use the graph in Figure 3.1 (created with a program available on the accompanying CD) which allows us to determine the post-test probability by drawing a line from the 50% pre-test probability to the post-test positive (+ve) line and across to the 86% post-test probability.

---

* The complement of this proportion describes the proportion of patients who do not have the target disorder and who have negative or normal test results [d/(c + d)]; this is called "specificity".

† The post-test odds are 0.45 × 6 = 2.7, and the post-test probability is 2.7/3.7 = 73%. Note that this is identical to the positive predictive value.

Extremely high values of sensitivity and specificity are useful, but not for the reasons you may think. When a test has a very high sensitivity (such as the loss of retinal vein pulsation in increased intracranial pressure), a negative result (the presence of pulsation) effectively rules out the diagnosis (of raised intracranial pressure). One of our clinical clerks suggested that we apply the mnemonic "SnNout" to such findings: when a sign has a high sensitivity (Sn), a negative (N) result rules out (out) the diagnosis. Similarly, when a sign has a very high specificity (Sp), such as the face of a child with Down's syndrome, a positive (P) result effectively rules in (in) the diagnosis (of Down's); not surprisingly, our clinical clerks call such a finding a "SpPin". We've listed some SpPins and SnNouts in Table 3.4, and have generated a longer list on our website (www.cebm.utoronto.ca). A perfect test would be both a SpPin and a SnNout (please let us know if you find one!). A useless test is one that leaves the probabilities unchanged (and the post-test lines both lie on the diagonal of the pre-test/post-test graph), which occurs when the sensitivity (%) + specificity (%)–100% (known as the Youden index) is zero.

We can generate likelihood ratios directly, or by reference to the sensitivity and specificity using formulae in Table 3.3:

The likelihood ratio for a positive test result is
$$LR+ = \text{sensitivity}/(1 - \text{specificity})$$

The likelihood ratio for a negative test result is
$$LR- = (1 - \text{sensitivity})/\text{specificity}$$

CAN I APPLY THIS VALID, IMPORTANT DIAGNOSTIC TEST TO A SPECIFIC PATIENT?

Having found a valid systematic review or individual report about a diagnostic test, and having decided that its accuracy is sufficiently high to be useful, how do we apply it to our patient? To transfer the study results, adapt them to our patient's unique pre-test probability, and decide this would be clinically useful, there are three questions we should ask; these are summarized in Table 3.5 and discussed below.

Table 3.4 Some SpPins and SnNouts[a]

Target disorder	SpPin (and specificity) [presence rules in the target disorder]	SnNout (and sensitivity) [absence rules out the target disorder]
Ascites (by imaging or tap)[b]	Fluid wave (92%)	History of ankle swelling (93%)
Pleural effusion[c]	Auscultatory percussion note loud and sharp (100%)	Auscultatory percussion note soft and/or dull (96%)
Increased intracranial pressure (by CT scan or direct measurement)[d]		Loss of spontaneous retinal vein pulsation (100%)
Cancer as a cause of lower back pain (by further investigation)[e]		Age >50 or cancer history or unexplained weight loss or failure of conservative therapy (100%)
Sinusitis (by further investigation)[f]		Maxillary toothache or purulent nasal secretion or poor response to nasal decongestants or abnormal transillumination or history of colored nasal discharge (LR = 0.1)
Alcohol abuse or dependency[g]	Yes to >3 of the CAGE questions (99.8%)	
Splenomegaly (by imaging)[h]	Positive percussion (Nixon method) and palpation	
Non-urgent cause for dizziness[i]	Positive head-hanging test and either vertigo or vomiting (94%)	

[a] To find more examples, and to nominate additions to the databank of SpPins and SnNouts, refer to this textbook's website at: <http://www.library.utoronto.ca/medicine/ebm/>.

[b] JAMA 1992; 267: 2645–8.

[c] J Gen Intern Med 1994; 9: 71–4.

[d] Arch Neurol 1978; 35: 37–40.

[e] JAMA 1992; 268: 760–5.

[f] JAMA 1993; 270: 1242–6.

[g] Am J Med 1987; 82: 231–5.

[h] JAMA 1993; 270: 2218–21.

[i] JAMA 1994; 271: 385–8.

Table 3.5 Questions to answer in applying a valid diagnostic test to an individual patient

1. Is the diagnostic test available, affordable, accurate, and precise in our setting?

2. Can we generate a clinically sensible estimate of our patient's pre-test probability?
   - From personal experience, prevalence statistics, practice data-bases, or primary studies?
   - Are the study patients similar to our own?
   - Is it unlikely that the disease possibilities or probabilities have changed since this evidence was gathered?

3. Will the resulting post-test probabilities affect our management and help our patient?
   - Could it move us across a test–treatment threshold?
   - Would our patient be a willing partner in carrying it out?
   - Would the consequences of the test help our patient reach his or her goals in all this?

1. Is the diagnostic test available, affordable, accurate, and precise in our setting?

We obviously can't order a test that is not available. Even if it is available, we may want to check around to be sure that it's performed and interpreted in a competent, reproducible fashion, and that its potential consequences (see below) justify its cost. For example, some of us work on medical units at more than one hospital and have found that the labs at these different hospitals use different assays for assessing ferritin D-dimer values, making the interpretation for clinicians more challenging! Moreover, diagnostic tests often behave differently among different subsets of patients, generating higher likelihood ratios in later stages of florid disease, and lower likelihood ratios in early, mild stages.

At least some diagnostic tests based on symptoms or signs lose power as patients move from primary care to secondary and tertiary care. Reference back to Table 3.3 can show you why. If patients are referred onward, in part because of symptoms, their primary care clinicians will be sending along patients in both cells "a" and "b", and subsequent evaluations of the accuracy of their symptoms will tend to show falling specificity due to the referral of patients with false-positive findings. If we think that any of these factors may be operating, we can try out what we judge to be clinically sensible variations in the likelihood ratios for the test result and see whether the results alter our post-test probabilities in a way that changes our diagnosis (the short-hand term for this sort of exploration is "sensitivity analysis").

2. Can we generate a clinically sensible estimate of our patient's pre-test probability?

This is a key topic, and deserves its own "section-within-a-section". How can we estimate our patient's pre-test probability? We've used five different sources for this vital information: clinical experience, regional or national prevalence statistics, practice databases, the original report we used for deciding on the accuracy and importance of the test, and studies devoted specifically to determining pre-test probabilities. Although the last is ideal, we'll take each in turn.

First, we can recall our clinical experience with prior patients who presented with the same clinical problem, and backtrack from their final diagnoses to their pre-test probabilities. While easily and quickly accessed, our memories are often distorted by our last patient, our most dramatic (or embarrassing) patient, our fear of missing a rare but treatable cause, and the like, so we use this source with caution.

And if we're early in our careers, we may not have enough clinical experience to draw upon. Thus, while we always use our remembered cases, we need to learn to supplement them with other sources, unless we have the time and energy to document all of our diagnoses and generate our own database.

Second, we could turn to regional or national prevalence statistics on the frequencies of the target disorders in the

---

* If you want to read more about how our minds and memories can distort our clinical reasoning, start with: Kassirer JP, Kopelman RI. Cognitive errors in diagnosis: instantiation, classification and consequences. Am J Med 1989; 86: 433–41.

general population or some subset of it. Estimates from these sources are only as good as the accuracy of their diagnoses, and, although they can provide some guidance for "baseline" pre-test probabilities before taking symptoms into account (useful, say, for patients walking into a general practice), we may be more interested in pre-test probabilities in just those persons with a particular symptom.

Third, we could overcome the foregoing problems by tracking down local, regional or national practice databases that collect patients with the same clinical problem and report the frequency of disorders diagnosed in these patients. Although some examples exist, such databases are mostly things of the future. As before, their usefulness will depend on the extent to which they use sensible diagnostic criteria and clear definitions of presenting symptoms.

Fourth, we could simply use the pre-test probabilities observed in the study we critically appraised for the accuracy and importance of the diagnostic test. If they really did sample the full spectrum of patients with the symptom or clinical problem (the second of our accuracy guides), we can extrapolate the pre-test probability from their study patients (or some subgroup of it) to our patient.

Fifth, and finally, we could track down a research report of a study expressly devoted to documenting pre-test probabilities for the array of diagnoses that present with a specific set of symptoms and signs similar to those of our patient. When done well, among patients closely similar to our patient, these studies provide the least biased source of pre-test probabilities for our use. Such studies are challenging to carry out, and one of us led the group who generated guides for their critical appraisal.[2] We've summarized these guides in Table 3.6. You'll see that most of them are already familiar to you, for they apply equally to reports of the accuracy and importance of diagnostic tests. We've provided examples of pre-test probabilities in Table 3.7, and will add to this list on our website (www.cebm.utoronto.ca).

1. Is this evidence about pre-test probability valid?

   - Did the study patients represent the full spectrum of those who present with this clinical problem?
   - Were the criteria for each final diagnosis explicit and credible?
   - Was the diagnostic work-up comprehensive and consistently applied?
   - For initially undiagnosed patients, was follow-up sufficiently long and complete?

2. Is this evidence about pre-test probability important?

   - What were the diagnoses and their probabilities?
   - How precise were these estimates of disease probability?

3. Will the resulting post-test probabilities affect our management and help our patient?

There are three elements of the answer to this final question and we begin with the bottom line: Could the test results move us across some threshold that would cause us to stop all further testing? Two thresholds should be borne in mind, as shown in Figure 3.3. First, if the diagnostic test was negative or generated a likelihood ratio down near 0.1, the post-test probability might become so low that we would abandon the diagnosis we were pursuing, and turn to other diagnostic possibilities. Put in terms of thresholds, this negative test result has moved us from above to below the "test threshold" in Figure 3.3 and we won't do any more tests for that diagnostic possibility. Second, if the diagnostic test came back positive or generated a high likelihood ratio, the post-test probability might become so high that we would also abandon further testing because we've made our diagnosis and would now move to choosing the most appropriate therapy; in these terms, we've now crossed from below to above the "treatment threshold" in Figure 3.3.

It is only if our diagnostic test result leaves us stranded between the test and treatment thresholds that we would continue to pursue that initial diagnosis by performing other tests. Although there are some very fancy ways of calculating test–treatment thresholds from test accuracy and the risks

Table 3.7 Examples of pre-test probabilities

Symptom or clinical problem	Source	Work-up	Disease probabilities
Anemia of chronic disease	90 adults admitted to a general medical ward of a county hospital in North America[a]	Clinical exam, blood testing, selected other testing	Infection, 36% Inflammation, 6% Malignant, 19% Renal, 15% Other, 24%
Dizziness >2 weeks	100 adult patients seen in primary care sites in one North American city[b]	Clinical exam, neurological, ophthalmologic, and psychological testing, selected other tests	Vertigo, 54% Psychiatric, 16% Multicausal, 13% Other, 19% Unknown, 8%
Dyspnea > 4 weeks, unexplained by exam, radiograph and spirometry	72 adults referred to outpatient pulmonary clinic in North America[c]	Standardized exam, testing and treatment	Respiratory, 36% Cardiac, 14% Hyperventilation, 19% Other, 12% Unexplained, 19%
Epilepsy, new onset in adults	333 adults presenting to a major urban emergency department in North America (excluded alcohol, head trauma, hypoglycemia)[d]	Standardized exam, testing (including head CT), and treatment	Unknown, 44% Stroke, 11% Tumor, 7% Infection, 17% Metabolic, 5% Other, 16%
Palpitations	190 patients from acute care sites in one North American city[e]	Clinical exam, cardiac and psychological testing, selected other tests	Cardiac, 43% Psychiatric, 31% Miscellaneous, 10% Unknown, 16%

[a] Am J Med 1989; 87: 638–44.
[b] Ann Intern Med 1992; 117: 898–904.
[c] Chest 1991; 100: 1293–9.
[d] Ann Emerg Med 1994; 24: 1108–14.
[e] Am J Med 1996; 100: 138–48.

Table 3.7 (cont'd)			
Symptom or clinical problem	Source	Work-up	Disease probabilities
Raynaud's pheno-menon	Literature review of published reports of secondary diseases in 639 patients with Raynaud's, from various settings[f]	Variable, usually clinical exam, selected serology and follow-up	Only 12.6% had or developed "secondary" disorders (e.g. systemic sclerosis, MCTD, SLE, etc.)

[f] Arch Intern Med 1998; 158: 595–600.

and benefits of correct and incorrect diagnostic conclusions,[*] intuitive test–treatment thresholds are commonly used by experienced clinicians and are another example of individual clinical expertise. We suggest you look at several pre-test scenarios using a post-test probability graph (Figure 3.1) to get a feel of when the test results in clinically useful shifts in decisions.

We may not cross a test–treatment threshold until we've performed several different diagnostic tests, and here is where another nice property of the likelihood ratio comes into play: provided the tests are independent we can "chain" the likelihood ratios. The post-test odds that result after the first diagnostic test we apply becomes the pre-test odds for our second diagnostic test. Hence we can simply keep multiplying the running product by the likelihood ratio generated from the next test. For example, when a 45-year-old man walks into our office, his pre-test probability of >75% stenosis of one or more of his coronary arteries is about 6%. Suppose that he gives us a history of atypical chest pain (only two of the three symptoms of substernal chest discomfort, brought on by exertion, and relieved in

---

* See the recommendations for additional reading, or: Pauker SG, Kassirer JP. The threshold approach to clinical decision-making. N Engl J Med 1980; 302: 1109.

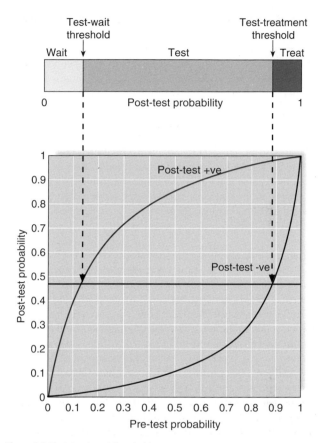

Figure 3.3 Test–treatment thresholds.

less than 10 minutes by rest are present, generating a likelihood ratio of about 13), and that his exercise ECG reveals 2.2 mm of non-sloping ST-segment depression (generating a likelihood ratio of about 11). Then his post-test probability for coronary stenosis is his pre-test probability (converted into odds) times the product of the likelihood ratios generated from his history[13] and exercise ECG,[11] with the resulting post-test odds converted back to probabilities (through dividing by its value +1), i.e.:

$(0.06/0.94) \times 13 \times 11 = 9.13$, and then $9.13/10.13 = 90\%$

The final result of these calculations is strictly accurate as long as the diagnostic tests being combined are "independent"; that is, given the "true" condition, the accuracy of one test does not further depend on another test. However, some dependence is common, and means we tend to over-estimate the informativeness of the multiple tests. Accordingly, we would want the calculated post-test probability at the end of this sequence to be comfortably above our treatment threshold before we would act upon it. This additional example of how likelihood ratios make lots of implicit diagnostic reasoning explicit is another argument in favor of seeking reports of overall likelihood ratios for sequences or clusters of diagnostic tests (see section on multiple tests below).

We should have kept our patient informed as we worked our way through all the foregoing considerations, especially if we've concluded that the diagnostic test is worth considering. If we haven't yet done so, we certainly need to do so now. Every diagnostic test involves some invasion of privacy, and some are embarrassing, painful, or dangerous. We'll have to be sure that the patient is an informed, willing partner in the undertaking. In particular, they should be aware of the possibility of false-positive or false-negative outcomes so that this is not a surprise when they return to discuss the results. The ultimate question to ask about using any diagnostic test is whether its consequences (reassurance when negative, labeling and possibly generating awful diagnostic and prognostic news if positive, leading to further diagnostic tests and treatments, etc.) will help our patient achieve his or her goals of therapy. Included here are considerations of how subsequent interventions match clinical guidelines or restrictions on access to therapy designed to optimize the use of finite resources for all members of our society.

MULTILEVEL LIKELIHOOD RATIOS

The more extreme a test result is, the more persuasive it is. Although the dichotomized serum ferritin sensitivity (90%) and specificity (85%) look impressive, expressing a test's accuracy with level-specific likelihood ratios reveals its even greater power and, in this particular example, shows how we can be misled by the restriction to just two levels (positive and negative) of the test result. Many test results, like serum ferritin, can be divided into several levels, and in Table 3.8 we show you a particularly useful way of dividing test results for ferritin into five levels.

When this is done, we see how much more informative extreme ferritin results are. The likelihood ratio for the "very positive" result is a huge 52, so that one extreme level of the test result can be shown to rule in the diagnosis, and in this case we can SpPin 59% (474/809) of the patients with iron deficiency anemia, despite the unimpressive sensitivity (59%) that would have been achieved if the ferritin results had been split just below this level. Likelihood ratios of 10 or more, when applied to pre-test probabilities of 33% or more $(0.33/0.67 = $ pre-test odds of 0.5) will generate post-test probabilities of $5/6 = 83\%$ or more.

Similarly, the other extreme level (>95) is a SnNout 75% (1332/1770) for those who do not have iron deficiency anemia (again despite a not-very-impressive specificity of 75%). Likelihood ratios of 0.1 or less, when applied to pre-test probabilities of 33% or less $(0.33/0.67 = $ pre-test odds of 0.5), will generate post-test probabilities of $0.05/1.05 = 5\%$ or less. The two intermediate levels (moderately positive and moderately negative) can move a 50% prior probability (pre-test odds of 1:1) to the useful but not necessarily diagnostic post-test probabilities of $4.8/5.8 = 83\%$ and $0.39/1.39 = 28\%$. The indeterminate level ("neutral") in the middle (containing about 10% of both sorts of patients) can be seen to be uninformative, with a likelihood ratio of 1. When diagnostic test results are around 1.0, we've learned nothing by ordering them. To give you a better "feel" for this, the impact of different likelihood ratios on different pre-test probabilities are shown in Figure 3.4. We've provided additional examples of likelihood ratios on this book's website (www.cebm.utoronto.ca).

Figure 3.4 can be used to do some approximate calculations. An easier way of manipulating all these calculations is the

Table 3.8 The usefulness of five levels of a diagnostic test result

Diagnostic test result	Serum ferritin (mmol/L)	Target disorder (Iron deficiency) present		Target disorder absent		Likelihood ratio	Diagnostic impact
		Number	%	Number	%		
Very positive	< 15	474	59 (474/809)	20	1.1 (20/1770)	52	Rule-in "SpPin"
Moderately positive	15–34	175	22 (175/809)	79	4.5 (79/1770)	4.8	Intermediate high
Neutral	35–64	82	10 (82/809)	171	10 (171/1770)	1	Indeterminate
Moderately negative	65–94	30	3.7 (30/809)	168	9.5 (168/1770)	0.39	Intermediate low
Extremely negative	≥ 95	48	5.9 (48/809)	1332	75 (1332/1770)	0.08	Rule-out "SnNout"
		809	100 (809/809)	1770	100 (1770/1770)		

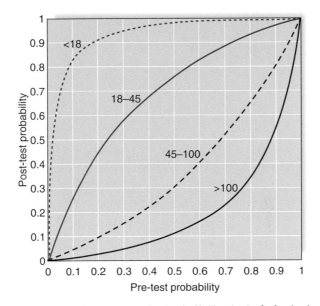

Figure 3.4 Probability revision graph using the likelihood ratios for four levels of ferritin.

nomogram of Figure 3.5 (also provided in the pocket cards that come with this book). You can check out your understanding of this nomogram by using it to replicate the results of Tables 3.3 and 3.8.

Now return to our patient with a pre-test probability for iron deficiency of 50% and a ferritin result of 60 mmol/L. To your surprise (we reckon!), our patient's test result generates an indeterminate likelihood ratio of only 1, and the test which we thought might be very useful, based on the old sensitivity and specificity way of looking at things, really hasn't been helpful in moving us toward the diagnosis. We'll have to think about other tests (including perhaps the reference standard of a bone marrow examination) to sort out her diagnosis.

More and more reports of diagnostic tests are providing multilevel likelihood ratios as measures of their accuracy. When their abstracts report only sensitivity and specificity,

Pre-test probability (%)	Likelihood ratio	Post-test probability (%)

Figure 3.5 A likelihood ratio nomogram.

we can sometimes find a table with more levels and generate our own set of likelihood ratios; at other times, we can find a scatterplot (of test results vs. diagnoses) that is good enough for us to be able to split them into levels.

MULTIPLE TESTS

Some reports of diagnostic tests go beyond even likelihood ratios, and one of their extensions deserves mention here. This extension considers multiple diagnostic tests as a cluster or sequence of tests for a given target disorder. These multiple results can be presented in different ways, either as clusters of positive/negative results or as multivariate scores, and in either case they can be ranked and handled just like other multilevel likelihood ratios. When they perform (nearly) as well in a second, independent ("test") set of patients, we often refer to them as "clinical prediction guides" (CPGs). In appraising the validity of a study of a CPG, we need to consider a 4th question in addition to those above:

Was the cluster of tests validated in a second, independent, group of patients?

Diagnostic tests are predictors, not explainers, of diagnoses. As a result, their initial evaluation cannot distinguish between real diagnostic accuracy for the target disorder and chance associations due to idiosyncrasies in the initial ("training" or "derivation") set of patients. This problem is compounded for clusters of diagnostic features (often called "clinical prediction guides"), where the large numbers of possible tests considered mean we may over-estimate the value of the few chosen in the CPG. The best indicator of accuracy in these situations is the demonstration of similar levels of accuracy when the test or cluster is evaluated in a second, independent (or "test"), set of patients. If it performs well in this "test" set, we are reassured about its accuracy. If it performs poorly, we should look elsewhere. And if no "test set" study has been carried out, we'd be wise to reserve judgment. CPGs are also used to help establish prognosis.

PRACTICING EBM IN REAL-TIME

CPGs often include several variables that we have to remember when trying to apply them to our patients. Several colleagues have attempted to make this easier and have provided interactive versions of clinical prediction guides available on websites; we've provided some of these on the accompanying website.

LEARNING AND TEACHING WITH CATS

Now that we have invested precious time and energy into finding and critically appraising an article, it would be a shame not to summarize and keep track of it so that we (and others) can use it again in the future. The means that Stephane Sauve, Hui Lee, and Mike Farkouh, residents on Dave Sackett's clinical service a few years ago, invented to accomplish this was to create a standardized one-page summary of the evidence organized as a "critically appraised topic", which they called a "CAT". We'll discuss these in more detail in Chapter 7, but note here that they provide a brief summary of the evidence that we can store for later retrieval. To help generate CATs, we've provided a copy of CATMaker on the CD, or it can be downloaded from the book's website (www.cebm.utoronto.ca) or from www.cebm.net. This software takes learners step by step through the creation of a CAT, calculates some of the clinically useful measures of therapy (NNTs, likelihood ratios), and automatically generates their confidence intervals. The CATMaker allows CATs to be saved (even in a draft "kitten" form that can be retrieved for later revision) or outputted in ".txt" files or ".html" formats. This means that you can create your own database to store your CATs in an easily retrievable format, make copies available to your students and colleagues, or even place them on your local intranet. Now take a look at the CAT we generated for ferritin.

SCREENING AND CASE-FINDING

So far, this chapter has focused on making a diagnosis for sick patients who have come to us for help. They are asking us to diagnose their ills and to help them as best we can, and only charlatans guarantee them longer life at the initial encounter. This final section of the chapter focuses on making early diagnoses of pre-symptomatic disease among well individuals in the general public (we'll call that "screening"), or among patients who have come to us for some other unrelated disorder (we'll call that "case-finding"). Individuals whom we might consider for screening and case-finding are not ill from the target disorders, so we are soliciting them with the promise (overt or covert) that they will live longer, or at least better, if they let us test them. Accordingly, the evidence we need about the validity of screening and case-finding goes beyond the accuracy of the

CAT Ferritin can diagnose iron deficiency in the elderly

> **Clinical bottom line** Serum ferritin can be very useful in diagnosing
> iron deficiency anemia in the elderly.

Clinical scenario. 75-year-old retired school-teacher (in for a check-up)
found to have an Hb of 100, with an MCV of 80, a negative history and
physical, and on no medications that are likely to suppress her marrow or
cause a bleed. I think her probability of iron deficiency is 1 out of 2 or 50%.

Three-part question. In an elderly symptomless woman with mild anemia,
would a serum ferritin help determine whether her bone marrow iron
stores were depleted?

Search terms. Searching *ACP Journal Club* using the terms "iron deficiency
anemia" and "ferritin", we find a study that appears to be of interest and
that provides a link to an overview of this topic.

The study

Independent...?	Yes
Blind...?	Yes
Standard applied regardless of test result...?	Yes
Appropriate spectrum...?	Can't tell

Target disorder and gold standard. **Bone marrow, stained for iron.**

Patients. Consecutive anemic patients in several inpatient and outpatient
settings. Transfused patients excluded.

Diagnostic test. Serum ferritin by radioimmunoassay.

The evidence

Test result	Present		Absent		
	No.	Prop.	No.	Prop.	LR
<15	474	0.59	20	0.01	51.85
15–34	175	0.22	79	0.04	4.85
35–64	82	0.10	171	0.11	1.05
65–94	30	0.04	168	0.09	0.39
≥95	48	0.06	1332	0.75	0.08

Comments
1. For elderly patients with symptomless anemia, go to the CT on anemia
   in the elderly to determine the yields from upper and lower
   gastrointestinal investigations.
2. Lots of labs are very slow in returning ferritin requests.

Expiry date: 2005.

References

Guyatt G H, Oxman A D, Ali M, et al. Laboratory diagnosis of iron deficiency
anemia: an overview. J Gen Intern Med 1992; 7: 45–53.

Patterson C, Guyatt G H, Singer J, et al. Iron deficiency in the elderly: the
diagnostic process. CMAJ 1991; 144: 435–40.

test for early diagnosis; we need hard evidence that patients are better off, in the long run, when such early diagnosis is achieved.

All screening and case-finding, at least in the short-run, harms some people. Early diagnosis is just that: people are "labeled" as having, or as being at high risk for developing, some pretty awful diseases (breast cancer, stroke, heart attack, and the like). And this labeling takes place months, years, or even decades before the awful diseases will become manifest as symptomatic illness (often in only a small portion of those who screen positive). Labeling hurts. For example, a cohort of working men studied both before and after they were labeled hypertensive displayed increased absenteeism, decreased psychological well-being, and progressive loss of income in comparison to their normotensive workmates (and these bad effects could not be blamed on drug side-effects, for they occurred even among men who were never treated!).[3] What's even worse is that those with false-positive screening tests will experience only harm (regardless of the efficacy of early treatment). But even individuals with true-positive tests who receive efficacious treatment have had "healthy time" taken away from them; early diagnosis may not make folks live longer, but it surely makes all of them "sick" longer!

We've placed this discussion at the end of the chapter on diagnosis, with the chapter on therapy the next but one, on purpose. In order to decide whether screening and case-finding do more good than harm, we'll have to consider the validity of claims about both the accuracy of the early diagnostic test and the efficacy of the therapy that follows it. We've summarized the guides for doing this in Table 3.9. Its elements are discussed in greater detail elsewhere (consult the "Further reading" at the end of this chapter).

1. Is there RCT evidence that early diagnosis really leads to improved survival, or quality of life, or both?

Earlier detection will always appear to improve survival. The "lead time" (between screen and usual detection; Figure 3.6) is always added to your apparent survival whether or not

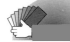

Table 3.9 Guides for deciding whether a screening or early diagnostic maneuver does more good than harm

1. Is there RCT evidence that early diagnosis really leads to improved survival, or quality of life, or both?
2. Are the early diagnosed patients willing partners in the treatment strategy?
3. How do benefits and harms compare in different people and with different screening strategies?
4. Do the frequency and severity of the target disorder warrant the degree of effort and expenditure?

there is any real change. Follow-up studies of placebo groups in randomized controlled trials (RCTs) have taught us that patients who faithfully follow health advice (by volunteering for screening or by taking their medicine) are destined for better outcomes before they begin. And, early diagnostic maneuvers preferentially identify patients with slower progressing, more benign disease. As a result, the only evidence we can trust in determining whether early diagnosis does more good than harm is a true experiment in

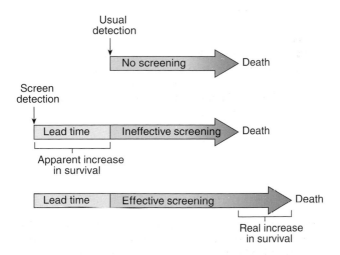

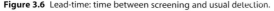

Figure 3.6 Lead-time: time between screening and usual detection.

which individuals were randomly assigned. As shown in Figure 3.7, this may be: (1) randomization to either undergo the early detection test (and, if truly positive, treated for the target disorder), or to be left alone (and only treated if and when symptomatic disease develops); or (2) be screened, and positives randomized to early treatment or usual care. The latter sort of evidence has been used for showing the benefits (and harms) of detecting raised blood pressure and cholesterol. The former sort of evidence showed the benefit of mammography for reducing deaths from breast cancer,* and showed the uselessness (indeed, harm) of chest X-rays for lung cancer. Ideally, their follow-up will consider functional and quality-of-life outcomes as well as mortality and discrete clinical events, and we should not be satisfied when the only favorable changes are confined to "risk factors".

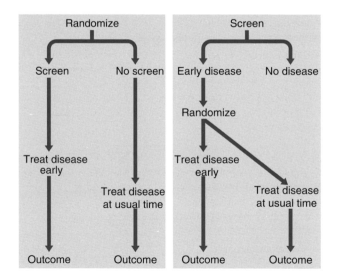

Figure 3.7 Two structures for randomized trials of the effectiveness of screening.

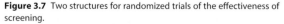

---

* Because only about a third of women whose breast cancers are diagnosed early go on to prolonged survival, even in this case the majority of positive screenees are harmed, not helped, by early detection.

2. Are the early diagnosed patients willing partners in the treatment strategy?

Even when therapy is efficacious, patients who refuse or forget to take it cannot benefit from it and are left with only the damage produced by labeling. Early diagnosis will do more harm than good to these patients, and we forget the magnitude of this problem at their peril (even by self-report, only half of patients describe themselves as "compliant"). There are quick ways of diagnosing low compliance and we'll show them to you in Chapter 5 (they comprise looking for non-attendance and non-responsiveness, and by non-confrontational questioning), but this is a diagnosis that you need to establish before, not after, you carry out any screening or case-finding.

3. How do benefits and harms compare in different people and with different screening strategies?

4. Do the frequency and severity of the target disorder warrant the degree of effort and expenditure?

This question raises, at the levels of both our individual practice and our community, the unavoidable question of rationing. Is going after the early diagnosis of this condition worth sacrificing the other good we could accomplish by devoting our own or our town's resources to some other purpose?

We don't want to sound too gloomy here, and won't leave this topic without pointing you to places where you can find some of the triumphs of screening and case-finding. A good place to start is the Canadian Task Force on the Periodic Health Examination, where there are some rigorously evaluated ones.[4]

TIPS FOR TEACHING AROUND DIAGNOSTIC TESTS

We usually begin by asking learners why we perform diagnostic tests, because they often respond: "To find out what's wrong with the patient [dummy!]". This provides an opening for helping them to recognize that diagnosis is not about finding absolute truth but about limiting uncertainty, and establishes both the necessity and the logical base for introducing probabilities, pragmatic test–treatment thresholds, and the like. It's also a time to get them to start thinking about what they're going to do with the results of the diagnostic test and about whether doing the test will really help their patient (maybe they'll conclude that the test isn't necessary!). A useful sequence is to elicit some disagreement between students (e.g. about a measurement or sign), but don't step in and suggest a "right" answer. The elicited disagreement can be used as an opening to unreliability and uncertainty. Comparison to a "gold standard" can introduce the issues of validity. While the formal calculations can be difficult, the qualitative ideas of SpPin and SnNout can be used, then be introduced to start students thinking about the accuracy and utility of a test.

When teaching about early diagnosis, we often challenge our learners with the statement "Even when therapy is worthless, early diagnosis always improves survival!", and then help them recognize the distortions that arise from drawing conclusions about volunteers, from starting survival measurements unfairly early in screened patients, and from failing to recognize that early detection tests preferentially identify slowly—rather than rapidly—progressive disease. Once they've grasped those ideas, we think they're safe from the evangelists of early diagnosis.

REFERENCES

1 Fleming KA. Evidence-based pathology. Evid Based Med 1997; 2: 132.

2 Guyatt GH, Rennie D, eds. Users' Guides to the Medical Literature. A Manual for Evidence-Based Clinical Practice. Chicago: AMA Press, 2002.

3 Macdonald LA, Sackett DL, Haynes RB, Taylor DW. Labelling in hypertension: a review of behavioural and psychological consequences. J Chron Dis 1984; 37: 933–42.

4 Canadian Task Force on the Periodic Health Examination. The periodic health examination. CMAJ 1979; 121: 1193–254.

Further reading

Guyatt GH, Rennie D, eds. Users' Guides to the Medical Literature. A Manual for Evidence-Based Clinical Practice. AMA Press: Chicago, 2002.

McGinn T, Randolph A, Richardson S, Sackett D. Clinical prediction guides. Evidence-Based Medicine 1998; 3: 5–6.

Sackett DL, Haynes RB, Guyatt GH, Tugwell P. Clinical Epidemiology: A Basic Science for Clinical Medicine, 2nd edn. Boston: Little, Brown, 1991, Ch. 4 (Interpretation of diagnostic data), Ch. 5 (Early diagnosis)

Whether posed by our patients, colleagues or ourselves, we frequently need to consider questions about prognosis. For example, a patient newly diagnosed with Alzheimer's dementia might ask, "What's going to happen to me?" As clinicians, we might consider: Should we screen for microalbuminuria in a patient with diabetes mellitus? Should a patient with microalbuminuria be treated with an angiotensin-converting enzyme inhibitor and will this change his prognosis? Recently, we were asked to consider the question: Should we screen asymptomatic astronauts for patent foramen ovale (What is the fate of an undetected patent foramen ovale during space flight?).

4

In order to answer these questions, and to make judgments about when to start and stop treatment, we need to evaluate evidence about prognosis for its validity, importance and relevance to our patients. The guides in Table 4.1 will help us tackle these issues. We'll consider the following clinical scenario to illustrate our discussion.

CLINICAL SCENARIO

We see a 45-year-old woman for a routine health visit who has recently moved to the city and enrolled in our practice. She is well and is on no medications. Her past medical history is unremarkable. On cardiac examination, auscultatory findings are suggestive of mitral valve prolapse with mitral regurgitation. The remainder of the examination, including heart rate, is unremarkable. On further questioning, the patient states that she's been told by a previous family physician that she has a heart murmur. She asks us if she should be concerned about this murmur.

In response to this scenario, we posed the question: In a 45-year-old woman with asymptomatic mitral valve prolapse, what is the risk of a cardiac event or death? Using the Clinical Queries function of PubMed (and clicking on the filters "prognosis" and "specificity"), we were able to identify an article that might help us to answer this question.[1]

TYPES OF REPORTS ON PROGNOSIS

Several types of studies can provide information on the prognosis of a group of individuals with a defined problem or risk factor. The best evidence with which to answer our clinical question would come from a systematic review of prognosis studies. A systematic review that searches for and combines all relevant prognosis studies would be particularly useful for retrieving information about relevant patient subgroups. When assessing the validity of a systematic review, we'd need to consider the guides in Table 4.1 as well as those in Table 5.9. At this time, relevant systematic reviews of prognosis studies are rare and we'll focus the discussion in this chapter on individual studies.

Table 4.1 Is this evidence about prognosis valid?

1. Was a defined, representative sample of patients assembled at a common point in the course of their disease?
2. Was follow-up of study patients sufficiently long and complete?
3. Were objective outcome criteria applied in a "blind" fashion?
4. If subgroups with different prognoses are identified:
   - Was there adjustment for important prognostic factors?
   - Was there validation in an independent group of "test-set" patients?

Cohort studies (in which investigators follow one or more groups of individuals with the target disorder over time and monitor for occurrence of the outcome of interest) represent the best design for answering prognosis questions. Randomized trials can also serve as a source of prognostic information (particularly since they usually include detailed documentation of baseline data), although trial participants may not be entirely representative of the population with a disorder. Case–control studies (in which investigators retrospectively assess prognostic factors by determining the exposures of cases who have already suffered the outcome of interest and controls who have not) are particularly useful when the outcome is rare or the required follow-up is long. However, the strength of inference that can be drawn from these studies is limited because of the potential for selection and measurement bias as discussed in Chapter 6.

Arriving at a diagnosis or prognosis rarely relies on a single sign, symptom, or laboratory test. Occasionally, when completing our literature search, we find articles describing tools that quantify the contributions that the clinical exam, laboratory, and radiological investigations make in establishing a diagnosis or a prognosis for a patient. These tools that combine diagnostic and prognostic information are called "clinical prediction guides" (CPGs), and are more fully discussed in Chapter 3.

ARE THE RESULTS OF THIS PROGNOSIS STUDY VALID?
1. Was a defined, representative sample of patients assembled at a common point in the course of their disease?
Ideally, the prognosis study we find would include the entire population of patients who ever lived who developed the disease, studied from the instant it developed. Unfortunately, this is impossible and we'll have to determine how close the report we've found is to the ideal with respect to how the target disorder was defined and how participants were assembled. If the study sample fully reflects the spectrum of illness we find in our own practice, we are reassured. However, considering our clinical scenario, if the study that we found included only patients from a specialty cardiology practice, we might not be satisfied that the sample is representative of the patients that we're interested in. The study should also describe the standardized criteria that were used to diagnose the target disorder.

But from what point in the disease should patients be followed? If investigators begin tracking outcomes only after some patients have already finished their course with the disease, then the outcomes for these patients might never be counted. Some would have recovered quickly, while others might have died quickly. So, to avoid missing outcomes by "starting the clock" too late, we look to see that study patients were included at a uniformly early time in the disease, ideally when it first becomes clinically manifest; this is called an "inception cohort". A study that assembled patients at any defined, common point in their disease may provide useful information if we want information only about that stage of the disease. However, if observations were made at different points in the course of disease for various people in the cohort, the relative timing of outcome events would be difficult to interpret. For example, it would be difficult to interpret the results from a study designed to determine the prognosis of patients with rheumatoid arthritis that included patients with newly diagnosed disease as well as those who had had the disease for 10 years or more. Ideally, we'd like to find a study in which participants are all at a similar stage in the course of the same disease.

Information about the study type and sampling method is usually found in the abstract and methods sections of the article. The study that we found is an inception cohort including patients with asymptomatic mitral valve prolapse.

2. Was the follow-up of the study patients sufficiently long and complete?

Ideally, every patient in the cohort would be followed until they fully recover or develop one of the disease outcomes. If follow-up is short, it may be that too few patients develop the outcome of interest and therefore we wouldn't have enough information to help us when advising our patients, and in this case we'd better look for other evidence. In contrast, if after years of follow-up, only a few adverse events have occurred, this good prognostic result is very useful in reassuring our patients about their future.

The more patients who are unavailable for follow-up, the less accurate the estimate of the risk of the outcome will be. The reasons for their loss are crucial. Some losses to follow-up are both unavoidable and mostly unrelated to prognosis (e.g. moving away to a different job) and these are not a cause for worry, especially if their numbers are small. But other losses might arise because patients die or are too ill to continue follow-up (or lose their independence and move in with family), and the failure to document and report their outcomes will reduce the validity of any conclusion the report draws about their prognosis.

Short of finding a report that kept track of every patient, how can we judge whether follow-up is "sufficiently complete"? There is no single answer for all studies, but we offer some suggestions to help. An analysis showing that the baseline demographics of the patients who were lost to follow-up are similar to those followed up provides some reassurance that certain types of participants were not selectively lost, but such an analysis is limited by those characteristics that were measured at baseline. Investigators cannot control for unmeasured traits that may be important prognostically, and that may have been more or less prevalent in the lost participants than in the followed-up participants. We suggest considering the simple "5 and 20" rule: fewer than 5% loss probably leads to little bias, greater than 20% loss seriously threatens validity, and in-between amounts cause intermediate amounts of trouble. While this may be easy to remember, it may over-simplify clinical situations in which the outcomes are infrequent. Alternatively, we could consider the "best" and "worst" case scenarios in an approach that we'll call a "sensitivity analysis". Imagine a study of prognosis wherein 100 patients enter the study, 4 die and 16 are lost to follow-up. A "crude" case-fatality rate would count the 4 deaths among the 84 with full follow-up, calculated as $4/84 = 4.8\%$. But what about the 16 who are lost? Some or all of them might have died too. In a "worst case" scenario, all would have died, giving a case-fatality rate of (4 known + 16 lost) = 20 out of (84 followed + 16 lost) = 100, or $20/100$ (i.e. 20%), which is four times the original rate that we calculated! Note that, for the "worst case" scenario, we've added the lost patients to both the numerator and the denominator of the outcome rate. On the other hand, in the "best case" scenario, none of the lost 16 would have died, yielding a case-fatality rate of 4 out of (84 followed + 16 lost), or 4/100 (i.e. 4%). Note that, for the "best case" scenario, we've added the missing cases to just the denominator. While this "best case" of 4% may not differ much from the observed 4.8%, the "worst case" of 20% does differ meaningfully, and we'd probably judge that this study's follow-up was not sufficiently complete and threatens the validity of the study. By using this simple sensitivity analysis, we can see what effect losses to follow-up might have on study results, which can help us judge whether the follow-up was sufficient to yield valid results.

> In the study that we found, follow-up was 97% at a median of 5.4 years, so no threat to validity here!

3. Were objective outcome criteria applied in a blind fashion?

Diseases affect patients in many important ways; some are easy to spot and some are more subtle. In general, outcomes at both extremes—death or full recovery—are relatively easy to detect with validity, but assigning a cause of death is often subjective (as anyone who has completed a death certificate knows!). In between these extremes are a wide range of outcomes that can be more difficult to detect or confirm, and where investigators will have to use judgment in deciding how to count them (e.g. readiness for return to work, or the intensity of residual pain). To minimize the effects of bias in measuring these outcomes, investigators should have established specific criteria to define each important outcome and then used them throughout patient follow-up. We'd want to satisfy ourselves that they are sufficiently objective for confirming the outcomes we're interested in. The occurrence of death is objective, but judging the underlying cause of death is very prone to error (especially when it's based on death certificates), and can be biased unless objective criteria are applied to carefully gathered clinical information. But even with objective criteria, some bias might creep in if the investigators judging the outcomes also know about the patients' prior characteristics. Blinding is crucial if any judgment is required to assess the outcome because unblinded investigators may search more aggressively for outcomes in people with the characteristic(s) felt to be of prognostic importance than in other individuals. In valid studies, investigators making judgments about clinical outcomes are kept "blind" to these patients' clinical characteristics and prognostic factors.

> In the mitral valve prolapse study that we found, the outcomes included total mortality and cause of death. Cause of death was ascertained by hospital notes, death reports, death certificates, and autopsy records, or by contacting the patients' physicians. It is not clear if the outcomes assessors were blinded.

4. If subgroups with different prognoses are identified, was there adjustment for important prognostic factors and validation in an independent "test set" patients?

Prognostic factors are demographic (e.g. age, gender), disease-specific (e.g. mitral valve prolapse with mitral regurgitation), or comorbid (e.g. hypertension) variables that are associated with the outcome of interest. Prognostic factors need not be causal—and in fact they are often not— but they must be strongly associated with the development of an outcome to predict its occurrence. For example, although mild hyponatremia does not cause death, serum sodium is an important prognostic marker in congestive heart failure (individuals with congestive heart failure and hyponatremia have higher mortality rates than heart failure patients with normal serum sodium).[2]

Risk factors are often considered distinct from prognostic factors, and include lifestyle behaviors and environmental exposures that are associated with the development of a target disorder. For example, smoking is an important risk factor for developing lung cancer, but tumor stage is the most important prognostic factor in individuals who have lung cancer.

Often we will want to know whether subgroups of patients have different prognoses (for example, among patients with mitral valve prolapse are those with moderate-to-severe mitral regurgitation or atrial fibrillation at increased risk of cardiovascular event or death compared with people without these findings). If a study reports that one group of patients had a different prognosis than another, first we need to see if there was any adjustment for known prognostic factors. By this we mean, did the authors make sure that these subgroup predictions are not being distorted by the unequal occurrence of another, powerful prognostic factor (such as would occur if patients with moderate-to-severe mitral regurgitation or atrial fibrillation were also more likely to have had a prior cardiac event than patients without these findings). There are both simple (e.g. stratified analyses displaying the prognoses of patients with mitral regurgitation separately for those with and without prior cardiac event) and fancy (e.g. multiple regression analyses that can take into account not only prior cardiac event but also left ventricular function and the like) ways of adjusting for these other important prognostic factors. We can examine the methods and results sections to reassure ourselves that one of these methods has been applied before we tentatively accept the conclusion about a different prognosis for the subgroup of interest.

We say "tentatively" because the statistics of determining subgroup prognoses are all about prediction, not explanation. They are indifferent to whether the prognostic factor is physiologically logical or a biologically nonsensical and random, non-causal quirk in the data (whether the patient lives on the north or the south side of the street, or was born under a certain astrological sign). For this reason, the first time a prognostic factor is identified, there is no guarantee that it really does predict subgroups of patients with different prognoses—it could be the result of a chance difference in its distribution between patients with different prognoses. Indeed, if investigators were to search for multiple potential prognostic factors in the same data set, a few would be likely to emerge on the basis of chance alone. The initial patient group in which prognostic factors are found is called a "training set" or "derivation set". Because of the risk of spurious, chance nomination of prognostic factors, we should look to see whether the predictive power of such factors has been confirmed in subsequent, independent groups of patients, termed "test sets" or "validation sets". To see if this was done, we'd look for a statement in the study's methods section describing a pre-study intention to examine this specific group of prognostic factors, based on their appearance in a training set or previous study. If a second, independent study validates the predictive power of prognostic factors, we have a very useful CPG of the sort that we met earlier in this section and which were discussed fully in Chapter 3, but this time predicting our patient's outcome after he or she is diagnosed.

> In our study, after adjusting for age, sex, and comorbid conditions, moderate-to-severe mitral regurgitation and ejection fraction <50% were found to be independent predictors of cardiovascular mortality. The authors also identified several prognostic factors that independently predicted cardiovascular morbidity and mortality. The significance of these prognostic factors was not confirmed in a validation set.

If the evidence about prognosis appears valid after considering the above guides, we can turn to examining its importance and applicability. But if we answered "no" to the questions above, we'd be better off searching for other evidence.

IS THIS VALID EVIDENCE ABOUT PROGNOSIS IMPORTANT? (TABLE 4.2)

Table 4.2 Is this valid evidence about prognosis important?
1. How likely are the outcomes over time?
2. How precise are the prognostic estimates?

1. How likely are the outcomes over time?

Once we're satisfied that an article's conclusions are valid, we can examine it further to see how likely each outcome is over time. Typically, results from prognosis studies are reported in one of three ways: as a percentage of survival at a particular point in time (such as 1-year or 5-year survival rates); as median survival (the length of follow-up by which 50% of study patients have died); or as survival curves that depict, at each point in time, the proportion (expressed as a percentage) of the original study sample who have NOT yet had a specified outcome. In prognosis studies we often find results presented as Kaplan–Meier curves, which are a type of survival curve.

Figure 4.1 shows four survival curves, each leading to a different conclusion. In panel A of this figure, virtually no patients have had events by the end of the study, which could mean that either prognosis is very good for this target disorder (in which case the study is very useful to us) or the study is too short (in which case this study isn't very helpful). In panels B, C and D, the proportion of patients surviving to 1 year (20%) is the same in all three graphs. And we could tell our patients that their chance of surviving for a year are 20%. However, the median survival (point at which half will have died—shown by the dashed line) is very different: 3 months for panel B, vs. 9 months for the disorder in panel C. The survival pattern is a steady, uniform decline only in panel D, and the median survival here is approximately 7.5 months. These examples highlight the importance of considering median survival and survival curves in order to fully inform our patient about prognosis.

2. How precise are the prognostic estimates?

As we pointed out earlier, investigators study prognosis in a sample of diseased patients, not the whole population of everyone who has ever had the disease. Purely by the play of chance, then, a study repeated 100 times among different groups of patients (even with identical entry characteristics) is bound to generate different estimates of prognosis. In deciding whether a given set of prognostic results is important, we need some means of judging just how much its results could vary by chance alone. The "confidence interval" provides the range of values that are likely to

Survival (%)

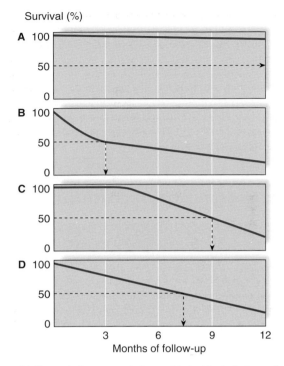

Figure 4.1 Prognosis shown as survival curves (dashed line indicates median survival). **A**: Good prognosis (or too short a study!). **B**: Poor prognosis early, then slower increase in mortality, with median survival of 3 months. **C**: Good prognosis early, then worsening, with median survival of 9 months. **D**: Steady prognosis.

include the true estimate, and quantifies the uncertainty in measurement. By convention, the "95% confidence interval" (95% CI) is used; this represents the range of values within which we can be 95% sure that the population value lies. The narrower the confidence interval, the more assured we can feel about the result. Note that, if survival over time is the outcome of interest, earlier follow-up periods usually include results from more patients than in later periods, so that survival curves are more precise (that is, they provide narrower confidence intervals) earlier in the follow-up. The text, tables or graphs of a good prognostic study include the confidence intervals for its estimates of prognosis (and if they don't, you ought to be able to apply Appendix 1 of this book and calculate the confidence interval for at least one of them yourself).

> From our study, we found that, at a median follow-up of 5.4 years, mortality was 11.5%. Moderate-to-severe mitral regurgitation (hazard ratio 1.8, 95% CI 1.03 to 3.0) and ejection fraction <50% (hazard ratio 2.3, 95% CI 1.05 to 4.4) were independent predictors of cardiovascular mortality.

CAN WE APPLY THIS VALID, IMPORTANT EVIDENCE ABOUT PROGNOSIS TO OUR PATIENT? (TABLE 4.3)

Table 4.3 Can we apply this valid, important evidence about prognosis to our patient?

1. Is our patient so different from those in the study that its results cannot apply?
2. Will this evidence make a clinically important impact on our conclusions about what to offer or tell our patient?

1. Is our patient so different from those in the study that its results cannot apply?

This guide asks us to compare our patients with those in the article, using descriptions of the study sample's demographic and clinical characteristics. Inevitably, some differences will turn up, so how similar is similar enough? We recommend framing the question the other way: Are the study patients so different from ours that we should not use the results at all in making predictions for our patients? For most differences, the answer to this question is "no", and thus we can use the study results to inform our prognostic conclusions.

2. Will this evidence make a clinically important impact on our conclusions about what to offer or tell our patient?

Evidence regarding a person's prognosis is clearly useful for deciding whether or not to initiate therapy, for monitoring therapy that has been initiated, and for deciding which diagnostic tests to order. If, for example, the study suggests an excellent prognosis for patients with a particular target disorder who didn't receive treatment, our discussions with patients would reflect these facts and would focus on whether any treatment should be started. If, on the other hand, the evidence suggests that the prognosis is gloomy without treatment (and if there are treatments that can make a meaningful difference), then our conversations with patients would reflect these facts and more likely lead us to treatment. Even when the prognostic evidence does not lead to a treat/don't treat decision, valid evidence can be useful in providing patients and families with the information they want about what the future is likely to hold for them and their illness.

Returning to our patient, transthoracic echocardiography revealed mild mitral regurgitation and an ejection fraction of >65%. Given her age (<50 years) and the absence of the other prognostic factors identified in the study that we found, we can reassure our patient that she is considered "low risk" for cardiovascular morbidity and mortality, and that her outcome (with respect to mitral valve prolapse) will be similar to that of the general population.

After we've gone to the trouble of retrieving and appraising an article, sometimes it's nice to keep a copy of our appraisal. We've provided on the accompanying CD an abbreviated version of our appraisal that you can download to your PDA.

PRACTICING EBM IN REAL-TIME

Sometimes we can't find the answers to our questions in high-quality, pre-appraised evidence resources, so we must appraise the primary literature ourselves. After we've done this, it's useful to keep a copy of the appraisal in case the same question arises again. On the accompanying CD, we've provided the CATMaker software which you can use to make a record of your appraisal and then save it in your own database. We've found this software to be a useful teaching tool, although we don't use it routinely in clinical practice because it takes too long. Instead, we have developed an abbreviated version that allows us to quickly record our question, the main study details, the results, and any comments/concerns about the study. We can save this as a "Word" file for our PC or for our PDA. Using this tool, we can develop our own database of topics that we encounter in our own practice. We've provided this "CQ log" on the accompanying CD and you can download it to your PDA; you can use it to log your clinical questions and the answers to those you've managed to track down. But keep in mind that these should have an expiry date on them! If we have colleagues close by, we can even share the work and collaborate on these.

REFERENCES

1   Avierinos JF, Gersh BJ, Melton J, et al. Natural history of asymptomatic mitral valve prolapse in the community. Circulation 2002; 106: 1355–61.

2   Mettauer B, Rouleau JL, Bichet D, et al. Sodium and water excretion abnormalities in congestive heart failure: determinant factors and clinical implications. Ann Intern Med 1986; 105: 161–7.

Further reading

Guyatt G, Rennie D, eds. Users' Guides to the Medical Literature. A Manual for Evidence-Based Clinical Practice. Chicago: AMA Press, 2002.

Sackett DL, Haynes RB, Guyatt GH, Tugwell P. Clinical Epidemiology. A Basic Science for Clinical Medicine, 2nd edn. Boston: Little, Brown, 1991.

After retrieving evidence, we need to decide if it's valid and important before we can apply the evidence to our individual patients. The order in which we consider validity and importance depends on individual preference. We could start by appraising its validity, arguing that, if it isn't valid, who cares whether it appears to show a huge effect? Alternatively, we could determine its clinical importance, arguing that, if the evidence doesn't suggest a clinically important impact, who cares if it's valid? We can start with either question, so long as we remember to follow-up one favorable answer with the other question. To illustrate our discussion, we'll consider the following patient.

CLINICAL SCENARIO

A 75-year-old man is seen in our office after being discharged from hospital 2 weeks previously. During this admission he underwent a carotid endarterectomy after suffering a transient ischemic attack (TIA), and being diagnosed with significant carotid stenosis. His hospital stay was uncomplicated and his discharge medications included metoprolol 50 mg twice daily for hypertension and aspirin 81 mg daily. Today, he has brought us an article from the Internet describing the benefits of statins for stroke prevention and he wonders what this medication is and if he should take it. Our note from his last visit showed that his total cholesterol was 5 mmol/L, HDL-cholesterol was 2.0 mmol/L, and LDL-cholesterol was 2 mmol/L. His examination was unremarkable.

Based on this scenario, we posed the following question: In a patient with history of TIA, carotid endarterectomy, hypertension, and normal lipid profile, does therapy with a statin decrease risk of stroke? Using PubMed Clinical Queries (see Ch. 2 for a description of this search engine)

5

we identified the recent MRC trial[1] which might help us answer this question. (We also found the MRC trial in *ACP Journal Club* online.)

TYPES OF THERAPEUTIC REPORTS

In this chapter we will initially tackle how to assess evidence about therapy from individual studies. However, individual trials are not the best evidence that we can find about the effects of therapy; ideally, we should seek an overview that systematically searches for and combines evidence from all trials relevant to the therapeutic topic, because this will provide us with a more reliable answer to our clinical question than the results from a single trial. For this reason, we suggested in Chapter 2 that our literature searches should always begin with looking for systematic reviews; the guides for determining their validity are given in Table 5.9. However, because systematic reviews assess their component trials individually (and because we want to be sure that they've done so in a valid way), and since at this point in time we're more likely to find individual trials than systematic reviews, we'll begin with discussing the individual trial. Sometimes the trial(s) will be insufficient by themselves for decision-making, and extrapolation or a detailed examination of the trade-offs between the benefits and harms of the intervention might be warranted. Also, our literature search might be extended to find a clinical decision analysis; rules for deciding whether it's valid are presented in Table 5.15. Similarly, we may want to track down an economic analysis; questions that will help us decide whether we can believe the results are listed in Table 5.18. Clinical practice guidelines outline evidence about diagnosis, prognosis, and therapy for a particular target disorder; guides for helping us decide if we want to apply them are given in Table 5.23. Qualitative studies can sometimes help guide us in our therapeutic decision-making; criteria to help us consider their validity are in Table 5.8. Finally, we may not be able to track down evidence that clearly helps us and our patients when making a decision about therapy; in these cases we might want to consider completing an "n-of-1" study (Table 5.25).

REPORTS OF INDIVIDUAL STUDIES

ARE THE RESULTS OF THIS INDIVIDUAL STUDY VALID?

> **Table 5.1** Is this evidence about therapy (from an individual randomized trial) valid?
>
> 1. Was the assignment of patients to treatment randomized?
> 2. Was the randomization concealed?
> 3. Were the groups similar at the start of the trial?
> 4. Was follow-up of patients sufficiently long and complete?
> 5. Were all patients analyzed in the groups to which they were randomized?
>
> Some finer points:
>
> 6. Were patients, clinicians, and study personnel kept blind to treatment?
> 7. Were groups treated equally, apart from the experimental therapy?

1. Was the assignment of patients to treatment randomized?

Until recently, it was believed that hormone replacement therapy (HRT) could decrease the risk of coronary artery disease (CAD) in post-menopausal women with a history of established CAD. This belief was based on data from several observational studies which found that women who used HRT had a decreased risk of the disease.[2] Clinicians and patients were subsequently surprised by the results of a randomized trial of women with established CAD, which found that the risk of CAD was not reduced with HRT![3] And, even more recently, the Women's Health Initiative study found that HRT was not effective in the primary prevention of CAD either.[4] Why such a difference between the results of the observational studies and the randomized trials? In observational studies, the patient's and/or physician's preferences determine whether or not the patient receives the treatment. Often, factors such as the presence of comorbid illnesses, use of other medications, and the severity of the disease and its symptoms influence the patient's and physician's therapeutic decision-making process. And, these same factors can also influence the risk of the outcome of interest (e.g. CAD). If these prognostic factors are unevenly distributed between treatment groups, this could exaggerate, cancel or even counteract the effects of therapy.*

Randomization balances the treatment groups for prognostic factors, even if we don't yet know enough about the target disorder to know what they all are. If these factors exaggerated the apparent effects of an otherwise ineffectual treatment, the effects of their imbalance could lead to the false-positive conclusion that the treatment was useful when in fact it wasn't. In contrast, if they nullified or counteracted the effects of a really efficacious treatment, this could lead to a false-negative conclusion that a useful treatment was useless or even harmful. We should insist on random allocation to treatment because it comes closer than any other research design to creating groups of patients at the start of the trial who are identical in their risk of the event we are trying to prevent. We need to determine if the investigators used some method analogous to tossing a coin† to assign patients to treatment groups (for example, the experimental treatment is assigned if the coin landed "heads", and a conventional, "control", or "placebo"‡ treatment is given if the coin landed "tails").

Randomization is something for investigators to be proud of, and often you'll find it mentioned explicitly in the abstract (or the title!). If the study wasn't randomized, we'd suggest that you stop reading it and go on to the next article in your search. (Note: We can begin to rapidly critically appraise articles by scanning the abstract to determine if the study is randomized; if it isn't, we can bin it.) Only if you can't find any randomized trials should you go back to it. If, however,

---

* Patient characteristics that are extraneous to the question posed and could cause the clinical outcome that we are trying to prevent with the treatment, and which might be unevenly distributed between the treatment groups, are called "confounders". Although there are other easy ways to avoid confounding (exclusion, stratified sampling, matching, stratified analysis, standardization, and multivariate modeling), they all require that we already know what the confounder is.

† In practice, this should be done by computers, but the principle remains the same.

‡ A placebo is a treatment that is so similar in appearance, taste, etc. to the active treatment that the patient, clinician, and study personnel cannot distinguish it.

the sole evidence you have about a treatment is from non-randomized studies, you have five options:

1. Check Chapter 2 again, or get some help in doing another literature search to see if you missed any randomized trials of the therapy.

2. See whether the treatment effect described in the non-randomized trial is so huge that you can't imagine it could be a false-positive study (this option is very rare, and usually only satisfied when the prognosis of untreated patients is uniformly terrible). As a check, you could ask your colleagues whether they consider the candidate therapy so likely to be efficacious that they'd consider it unethical to randomize a patient like yours into a study of it that includes a no-treatment or placebo group.

3. If the non-randomized trial concluded that the treatment was useless or harmful, then it is usually safe to accept that conclusion. False-positive conclusions from non-randomized studies are far more common than false-negative ones (since treatments are typically withheld from patients with the poorest prognoses, and patients who faithfully take their medicine are destined for better outcomes, even when they are taking worthless treatments or placebos!).

4. Consider whether an "n-of-1" trial would make sense to you and your patient (Table 5.25).

5. Try to find evidence for another management option.

> In the MRC trial that we found to answer our question about the effectiveness of statin therapy, the title states that it is a randomized trial, and a quick scan of the methods refers us to another article for complete details.

2. Was the randomization concealed?

We should look to see if randomization was concealed from the clinicians and study personnel who entered patients into the trial. If allocation was concealed, the clinicians would be unaware of which treatment the next patient would receive and thus unable, consciously or unconsciously, to distort the balance between the groups being compared. As with failure to use randomization, inadequate concealment of allocation can distort the apparent effect of treatment in either direction, causing the effect to seem larger or smaller than it really is. Often, articles don't state whether the randomization list was concealed, but if randomization occurred by telephone or by some system that was at a distance from where patients were being entered into the trial, we can be assured by this. (Allocation concealment will not be achieved by using transparent envelopes—even if they're sealed!)

3. Were the groups similar at the start of the trial?

We should check to see if the groups were similar in all prognostically important ways (except for receiving the treatment) at the start of the trial. As noted above, the benefit of randomization is the equal distribution of potential confounders between the study groups. However, baseline differences between the study groups may be present due to chance. If the groups aren't similar, we must determine if adjustment for these potentially important prognostic factors was carried out. It is reassuring if the adjusted and unadjusted analyses yield similar results.

> In the statin study, there were no significant differences between patients receiving placebo and those receiving statin.

4. Was follow-up of patients sufficiently long and complete?

Once we are satisfied that the study was randomized, we can look to see if all patients who were entered into the trial were accounted for at its conclusion. Ideally, we'd like to see that no patients were lost to follow-up because these patients may have had outcomes that would affect the conclusions of the study. If, for example, patients receiving the experimental treatment dropped out because of adverse outcomes, their absence from the analysis would lead to an over-estimation of the efficacy of the treatment.

What can we consider to be an acceptable loss? To be sure of a trial's conclusion, the investigators should be able to take all patients who were lost to follow-up, assign them the worst case outcome (assume that everyone lost from the group whose remaining members fared better had a bad outcome, and that everyone lost from the group whose remaining members fared worse had a good outcome), and still be able to support their original conclusion. If this method doesn't change the study's conclusions, the loss to follow-up is not a threat to the study's validity. However, if the study result does change, its validity is threatened and we must decide if the results derived from the worst case method are plausible. It would be unusual for a trial to withstand a worst case analysis if it lost more than 20% of its patients (but this depends on the number of outcomes observed; for example, if few outcomes were observed in a large study, the loss of 20% of patients could have a big impact on the results) and journals such as *Evidence Based Medicine* and *ACP Journal Club* won't publish trials with <80% follow-up.

We should also ensure that the follow-up of patients was sufficiently long to see a clinically important effect. For example, if our study assessing the use of statins only followed up patients for 1 week or 1 month, we wouldn't find the results very helpful. Given the nature of the target disorder, we'd like to see a follow-up period of several months or, ideally, years. Sometimes information about follow-up is available in the study's abstract, but most often we have to turn to the results to obtain specific details.

> In our statin study, follow-up was 99% at a mean of 5 years.

5. Were all patients analyzed in the groups to which they were randomized?

Because anything that happens after randomization can affect the chance that a study patient has the outcome of interest, it's important that all patients (even those who fail to take their medicine, or accidentally or intentionally receive the wrong treatment) are analyzed in the groups to which they were allocated; once comparable groups are set up at the study onset, they should stay this way in order to preserve randomization. It has been shown repeatedly that patients who "do" and "don't" take their study medicine have very different outcomes, even when the study medicine they have been prescribed is a placebo. The study participants that left the study or crossed over into another treatment group may have a particular characteristic, so that those remaining in the groups are no longer comparable as they were at the study onset. To preserve the value of randomization, we should demand an "intention-to-treat analysis" whereby all patients are analyzed in the groups to which they were initially assigned, regardless of whether they received their assigned treatment. It is important that we not only look for the term "intention-to-treat analysis" in the methods but also look at the results to ensure that this analysis was actually done.

> The statin study used an intention-to-treat analysis and we can feel confident that it has passed all major validity criteria.

6. Were patients, clinicians, and study personnel kept blind to treatment?

Blinding is necessary to avoid patients' reporting of symptoms or their adherence to treatment being affected by hunches about whether the treatment is effective. Similarly, blinding prevents the report or interpretation of symptoms from being affected by the clinician's or outcomes assessor's suspicions about the effectiveness of the study intervention. Not surprisingly, blinding is particularly important when the outcome of interest is subjective, and more judgment by the clinician or outcomes assessor is necessary.

When patients and clinicians can't be kept blind (such as in surgical trials), often it is possible to have other, blinded clinicians assess clinical records (purged of any mention of treatment) or to use objective outcome measurements. For example, in the North American Symptomatic Carotid Endarterectomy Trial[5] (this study randomized patients with symptomatic carotid stenosis to either carotid endarterectomy or medical therapy with aspirin), the patients in the surgical group could obviously not be blinded to the treatment they received. Outcome events were assessed by four groups: the participating neurologist and surgeon; the neurologist at the study center; "blinded" members of the steering committee; and "blinded" external adjudicators.

Of note, a recent study[6] has shown that clinicians interpret the term "double-blind" differently; ideally, an article should explicitly state who was blinded, but it is rare to find articles that do this. Information about blinding may be present in the abstract or the methods section (and sometimes the title) of the article.

> The MRC trial states that it was a double-blind placebo-controlled trial.

7. Were groups treated equally, apart from the experimental therapy?

Blinding of patients, clinicians and study personnel can prevent them from adding any additional treatments (or "co-interventions"), apart from the experimental treatment, to just one of the groups. Usually, we can find information about co-interventions in the methods and/or results sections of an article.

If the study fails any of the criteria discussed above, we need to decide if the flaw is significant and threatens the validity of the study. If this is the case, we'll need to look for another study. If we find that our article satisfies all of the criteria, we can proceed to consideration of its importance.

ARE THE VALID RESULTS OF THIS INDIVIDUAL STUDY IMPORTANT?

Table 5.2 Is this valid evidence about therapy (from an individual randomized trial) important?

1. What is the magnitude of the treatment effect?
2. How precise is the estimate of the treatment effect?

In this section, we'll discuss how to determine if the potential benefits (or harms) of the treatment described in a study are important. We'll refer to the guides in Table 5.2 for this discussion. Deciding whether we should be impressed with the results of a trial requires two steps: first, finding the most useful clinical expression of these results; and second, comparing these results with the results of other treatments for other target disorders.

1. What is the magnitude of the treatment effect?

There are a variety of methods that we can use to describe results; we've included the most important ones in Table 5.3, and we'll illustrate them with the help of the statin study. As you can see from the actual trial results in Table 5.3, at a mean of 5 years' follow-up, stroke occurred among 5.7% of patients randomized to the control group (we'll call this the "control event rate", CER), and in 4.3% of the patients assigned to receive statin therapy (we'll call this the "experimental event rate", EER). This difference was statistically significant, but how can it be expressed in a clinically useful way? Most often we see this effect reported in clinical journals as the relative risk reduction (RRR) calculated as ($|$CER − EER$|$/CER). In this example, the RRR is (5.7% − 4.3%)/5.7% (i.e. 25%), and we can say that statin therapy decreased the risk of stroke by 25% relative to those who received placebo. In a similar way, we can describe the situation in which the experimental treatment increases the risk of a good event as the "relative benefit increase" (RBI; also calculated as $|$CER − EER$|$/CER). Finally, if the treatment increases the probability of a bad event, we can use the same formula to generate the "relative risk increase" (RRI).

One of the disadvantages of the RRR, which makes it unhelpful for our purposes, is revealed in the hypothetical data outlined in the bottom row of Table 5.3. The RRR doesn't reflect the risk of the event without therapy (the CER, or baseline risk), and therefore cannot discriminate huge treatment effects from small ones. For example, if the stroke risk was trivial (0.000057%) in the control group and

Table 5.3 Measures of effect size

	Event rate = stroke (mean follow-up 5 years)		Relative risk reduction (RRR)	Absolute risk reduction (ARR)	Number needed to treat (NNT)
	Control rate (CER)	Experimental event rate (EER)	|CER − EER|/CER	|CER − EER|	1/ARR
MRC trial	5.7%	4.3%	|5.7% − 4.3%| /5.7% = 25%	|5.7% − 4.3%| = 0.014 or 1.4%	1/1.4% = 72
Hypothetical, trivial case	0.000057%	0.000043%	|0.000057% − 0.000043%| /0.000057% = 25%	|0.000057% − 0.000043%| = 0.0000014%	1/0.0000014% = 7142857

similarly trivial (0.000043%) in the experimental group, the RRR remains 25%!

One measure that overcomes this lack of discrimination between small and large treatment effects looks at the absolute arithmetic difference between the rates in the two groups. This is called the "absolute risk reduction" (ARR) (or the risk difference) and it preserves the baseline risk. In the statin trial, the ARR is 5.7% − 4.3% = 1.4%. In our hypothetical case where the baseline risk is trivial, the ARR is trivial too, at 0.000014%. Thus, the ARR is a more meaningful measure of treatment effects than is the RRR. When the experimental treatment increases the probability of a good event, we can generate the "absolute benefit increase" (ABI), which is also calculated by finding the absolute arithmetic difference in event rates. Similarly, when the experimental treatment increases the probability of a bad event, we can calculate the "absolute risk increase" (ARI).

The inverse of the ARR (1/ARR) is a whole number and has the useful property of telling us the number of patients that we need to treat (NNT) with the experimental therapy for the duration of the trial in order to prevent one additional bad outcome. In our example, the NNT is 1/1.4% = 72, which means we would need to treat 72 people with a statin (rather than placebo) for 5 years to prevent one additional person from suffering a stroke. In our hypothetical example, in the bottom row of Table 5.3, the clinical usefulness of the NNT is underscored, for this tiny treatment effect means that we would have to treat over 7 million patients for 5 years to prevent one additional bad event!

Should we be impressed with an NNT of 72? We can get an idea by comparing it with NNTs for other interventions and durations of therapy, tempered by our own clinical experience and expertise. The smaller the NNT is, the more impressive the result. However, we should also consider the seriousness of the outcome that we are trying to prevent. We've provided some examples of NNTs in Table 5.4. For example, we'd only need to treat 7 people with mild-to-moderate Alzheimer's dementia with donepezil to prevent

Table 5.4 Some useful NNTs[a]

Target disorder	Intervention	Events being prevented	Event rate		Follow-up time	NNT
			CER	EER		
Diastolic blood pressure 115–129 mmHg[b]	Antihypertensive drugs	Death, stroke, or MI	13%	1.4%	1.5 years	8
Diastolic blood pressure 90–109 mmHg[c]	Antihypertensive drugs	Death, stroke or MI	5.5%	4.7%	5.5 years	128
Symptomatic high-grade carotid stenosis[d]	Carotid endarterectomy (compared with medical therapy)	Death or major stroke	18%	8%	2 years	10
Mild-to-moderate Alzheimer's dementia[e]	Donepezil (vs. placebo)	No functional decline	44%	59%	1 year	7
Unstable angina[f]	Invasive management within 7 days (compared with medical management)	Death or MI	16%	12%	24 months	24
Renal insufficiency and undergoing coronary angiogram[g]	Oral acetylcysteine (vs. placebo)	Contrast media-induced reduction in renal function	12%	4%	48 hours	12

[a] See www.cebm.utoronto.ca for additional NNTs.
[b] JAMA 1967; 202: 116–22.
[c] BMJ 1995; 291: 97–104.
[d] N Engl J Med 1991; 325: 445–53.
[e] Neurology 2001; 57: 613–20.
[f] J Am Coll Cardiol 2002; 40: 1902–14.
[g] JAMA 2003; 289: 553–8.

one person from experiencing functional decline at 1 year. In contrast, we'd have to treat over 100 people with hypertension for 5.5 years to prevent one death, stroke or myocardial infarction. If you want to see more NNTs, visit our website (www.cebm.utoronto.ca) or take a look at the CD that accompanies this book; you can download some NNT tables to your PDA and nominate an NNT for inclusion on the website.

We can describe the adverse effects of therapy in an analogous fashion, as the number needed to cause harm to one more patient (NNH) from the therapy. The NNH is calculated as 1/ARI. In the statin study, 0.03% of the control group experienced rhabdomyolysis compared with 0.05% of patients who experienced this in the group that received a statin. This absolute risk increase of $|0.03\% - 0.05\%| = 0.02\%$ generates an NNH over 5 years of 5000. This means that we'd need to treat 5000 patients with a statin for 5 years to cause one additional patient to have rhabdomyolysis. Thus, the NNT and NNH provide us with a nice measure of the effort we and our patients have to expend to prevent or cause one more bad outcome, and their attractiveness as an effort:yield ratio (or "poor clinicians' cost-effectiveness analysis") is easily recognized.

To understand NNTs, we need to consider some additional features. First, they always have a dimension of follow-up time associated with them. Quick reference to Table 5.4 reminds us that the NNT of 10 to prevent one more major stroke or death by performing endarterectomy on patients with symptomatic high-grade carotid stenosis refers to outcomes over a 2-year period (in this case, from an operation that is over in minutes). One consequence of this time dimension is that, if we want to compare NNTs for different follow-up times, we have to make an assumption about them and a "time adjustment" to at least one of them. Say that we wanted to compare the NNTs to prevent one additional stroke, myocardial infarction or death with drugs among patients with mild vs. severe hypertension. Another quick look at Table 5.4 gives us an NNT at 1.5 years of just 8 for severe hypertensives (who already have a lot of target organ damage), and an NNT at 5.5 years of 128 for milder hypertensives (most of whom are free of target organ damage). To compare their NNTs, we need to adjust at least one of them so that they relate to the same follow-up time. The assumption that we make here is that the RRR from antihypertensive therapy is constant over time (i.e. we assume that antihypertensive therapy exerts the same relative benefit in year 1 as it does over the next 4 years). If we are comfortable with that assumption (it appears safe for hypertension), we can then proceed to make the time adjustment.

Let's adjust the NNT for the mild hypertensives (128 over the "observed" 5.5 years) to an NNT corresponding to a "hypothetical" 1.5 years. This is done by multiplying the NNT for the "observed" follow-up time by a fraction with the "observed" time in the numerator and the "hypothetical" time in the denominator. In this case, adjusting the NTT of 128 for mild hypertensives to its hypothetical value for 1.5 years becomes:

$$NNT_{hypothetical} = NNT_{observed} \times (observed\ time/$$
$$hypothetical\ time)$$
$$NNT_{1.5} = 128 \times (5.5/1.5) = 470$$

(By convention, we round any decimal NNT upwards to the next whole number.) Now we can appreciate the vast difference in the yield of clinical efforts to treat mild vs. severe hypertensives: we need to treat 470 of the former, but only 3 of the latter for 1.5 years in order to prevent one additional bad outcome. The explanation lies in the huge difference in CERs (far higher in severe hypertensives followed for just 1.5 years than in mild hypertensives followed for 5.5 years).

Second, returning to Table 5.3, we calculated an NNT of 72; but patients can have a different baseline risk of the outcome (depending on the presence of comorbid illnesses, etc.), and therefore they may be of higher or lower risk of the event than the "average" patient in the study. The NNT can be adjusted for our patient's individual baseline risk of the outcome; this will be discussed in detail on p. 134.

2. How precise is this estimate of the treatment effect?

The third thing we need to remember about the NNT is that, like any other clinical measure, NNTs are estimates of the truth and we should specify the limits within which we can confidently state that the true NNT lies. If we want to specify the limits within which the true NNT lies 95% of the time, it's called specifying the "95% confidence interval" (95% CI). The confidence interval provides the range of values that are likely to include the true risk and quantifies the uncertainty in measurement. For example, consider a hypothetical NNT of 72 with a 95% CI of 51 to 1170; we would have 95% confidence that the true NNT value lies between 51 and 1170. The smaller the number of patients in the study that generated the NNT, the wider its confidence interval, but, even when the confidence interval is wide, it can provide us with some guidance and we should look at the limits of the confidence interval. In our hypothetical example above, the trial shows a positive effect, but we need look at the upper limit of the confidence interval for the NNT. Is the value of 1170 clinically important? If we decide that it isn't, the study results are unhelpful even though it is statistically significant. Similarly, if the study results are negative, we can look at the limits of the confidence interval to see if a potentially important positive benefit has been excluded. If you'd like to read more about confidence intervals, we refer you to Appendix 1.

PRACTICING EBM IN REAL-TIME
Calculating the measures of treatment effect: a short-cut

Rather than memorizing the formula described above, we could instead use an EBM calculator whenever we need to calculate the measure of the treatment effect (i.e. if the results of the study aren't presented in the article using these measures). This tool saves us time and decreases the risk of a mathematical error. From our website and from the accompanying CD you can download an EBM calculator that we've developed (www.cebm.utoronto.ca); the calculator can also be downloaded to your PDA.

Let's try to repeat the calculations that we completed in Table 5.3. In the dropdown box on the calculator, click on the RCT (randomized clinical trial) option. We can enter the data from the table and at a click of a button we can obtain the measures of effect and their confidence intervals (see Figure 5.1).

Using pre-appraised evidence

When retrieving evidence, we also completed a search of *ACP Journal Club* and identified an entry for the MRC trial.[7] We know that this article has passed some quality filters since it appears in this journal (Ch. 2). Contrast this more informative abstract with that from the original article. We can quickly see that it was a randomized, placebo-controlled study in which patients, clinicians, data collectors, and outcomes assessors were blind. The investigators used an intention-to-treat analysis, and greater than 99% follow-up of patients was achieved over a mean of 5 years. Of note, a declarative title and the clinical question that the trial addressed (using the PICO format!) are included. Using the *ACP Journal Club* abstract, we can appraise the trial's validity

Address	http://www.cebm.utoronto.ca/dev/ebmccalc1_7/ebmcalc_v1_7.html

Diagnostic Test	Prospective Study	Case Control Study	**RCT**

Enter the data to the table below

	Outcome	No outcome
Experimental	442 a	b 9827
Control	585 c	d 9682

Clear Table	Get Results

Chi-squared: 20.697		p-value: <0.0001
	Estimate	**95% CI**
Relative Risk Reduction (RRR)	0.245	[0.148 to 0.33]
Absolute Relative Risk (ARR)	0.014	[0.008 to 0.02]
Number Needed to Treat (NNT)	71.754	[50 to 125]

Enter the following values below to calculate the Fully-adjusted LHH=(1/NNT) x f_t x s : (1/NNH) x f_h

f_t = Factor (treatment) [ ] f_h= Factor (harm) [ ]   s [ ]   Calculate

LHH =

Figure 5.1 Using the EBM calculator.

and importance in less than a minute and quickly move to decide if we can apply the evidence to our patient!

ARE THE VALID, IMPORTANT RESULTS OF THIS INDIVIDUAL STUDY APPLICABLE TO OUR PATIENT?

Now that we have decided that the evidence we have found is both valid and important, we need to consider if we can apply it to our own patient. To apply evidence, we need to integrate the evidence with our clinical experience and expertise, and with our patient's values and preferences. The guides for doing this are in Table 5.5.

1. Is our patient so different from those in the study that its results cannot apply?

We need to use our clinical expertise to decide if our patient is so different from those in the study that its results don't apply. One approach would be to demand that our patient fit all the inclusion criteria for the study and reject it if our patient doesn't fit each one. This isn't a very sensible approach because most differences between our patients and those in trials tend to be quantitative (they have different ages, or different degrees of risk of the outcome event, or different responsiveness to the therapy) rather than qualitative (total absence of responsiveness to treatment or risk of event). We'd suggest that a far more appropriate approach is to consider whether our patient's

Table 5.5 Is this valid and important evidence (from an individual randomized trial) applicable to our patient?

1. Is our patient so different from those in the study that its results cannot apply?

2. Is the treatment feasible in our setting?

3. What are our patient's potential benefits and harms from the therapy?

4. What are our patient's values and expectations for both the outcome we are trying to prevent and the treatment we are offering?

sociodemographic features or pathobiology are so different from those in the study that its results are useless to us and our patient; only then should we discard its results and resume our search for relevant evidence. There are only a few occasions when this might be the case: different pharmacogenetics, absent immune responses, comorbid conditions that prohibit the treatment, and the like. As a consequence of this clinical (as opposed to actuarial) approach, it's rare that we have to toss away a study for this reason. One difference we do need to consider is whether our patient is likely to accept our advice and comply with the demands of the therapeutic regimen; we'll address that at the end of this section.

Sometimes treatments appear to produce qualitative differences in the responses of subgroups of patients so that they appear to benefit some subgroups but not others. Such qualitative differences in response are extremely rare. For example, some early trials of aspirin for TIAs showed large benefits for men but none for women; subsequent trials and systematic reviews showed that this was a chance finding and that aspirin is efficacious in women. If you think that the treatment you're examining may work in a qualitatively different way among different subgroups of patients, you should refer to the guides in Table 5.6. To summarize them, unless the difference in response makes biological sense, was hypothesized before the trial, and has been confirmed in a second, independent trial, we'd suggest that you accept the treatment's overall efficacy as the best starting point for estimating its efficacy in your individual patient.

2. Is the treatment feasible in our setting?

Next, we need to consider if the treatment is feasible in our practice setting. Can our patient, or health care system pay for the treatment, its administration, and the required monitoring? Is the treatment available in our setting? Statin therapy is currently "free" for use with certain conditions in some regions and countries, but, in others, patients would be required to pay for it themselves.

> **Table 5.6** Guides for whether to believe apparent qualitative differences in the efficacy of therapy in some subgroups of patients
>
> A qualitative difference in treatment efficacy among subgroups is likely only when ALL the following questions can be answered "yes":
>
> 1. Does it really make biological and clinical sense?
> 2. Is the qualitative difference both clinically (beneficial for some but useless or harmful for others) and statistically significant?
> 3. Was it hypothesized before the study began (rather than the product of dredging the data)?
> 4. Was it one of just a few subgroup analyses carried out in the study?
> 5. Has the result been confirmed in other independent studies?

3. What are our patient's potential benefits and harms from the therapy?

After we have decided that the study is applicable to our patients and that the treatment is feasible, we need to estimate our patient's unique benefits and risks of therapy. There are two general approaches to doing this. The first, and longer, approach begins by coming up with the best possible estimate of what would happen to our patient if he were not treated: his individual CER or "patient's expected event rate" (PEER). To this estimate we can apply the overall RRR (for the events we hope to prevent with therapy) and RRI (for the adverse effects of therapy), and generate the corresponding NNT and NNH for our specific patient. The second, much quicker, approach skips this PEER step and works entirely from the NNT and NNH in the study. Note that, with both approaches, we assume that the relative benefits and risks of therapy are the same for patients with high and low PEERs. Because the second method is so much quicker, you might want to skip to p. 135, but if you want to learn the long way (first), read on.

The long way, via PEER

There are four ways to estimate our patient's PEER. First, we can simply assign our patient the overall CER from the study; this is easy, but sensible only if our patient is like the "average" study patient. Second, if the study has a subgroup of patients with characteristics similar to our own patient, we can assign to him the CER for that subgroup. (Indeed, in the unlikely event that we could say "yes" to all of the questions posed in Table 5.6, we could even apply the ARR for that subgroup to generate an NNT for our patient.) Third, if the study report includes a valid clinical prediction guide, we could use it to assign a PEER to our patient. Fourth, we could look for another paper that described the prognosis of untreated patients like ours and use its results to assign our patient a PEER. All four methods we've described generate a PEER for our patient—what we would expect to happen to them if they received the "control" or comparison intervention in the study we're using. To convert this into an NNT or NNH for patients just like ours, we have to apply the corresponding RRR and RRI to them, using the formula:

$$NNT = 1/(PEER \times RRR)$$

For example, suppose that we find a paper that suggests that our vascular patient has a risk of stroke of 30% over 5 years given his risk factors and comorbidities (so his PEER is 30%). The MRC trial generated an overall RRR of 25%, so the NNT for patients like ours is $1/(30\% \times 25\%) = 13$. Similarly, to calculate the NNH:

$$NNH = 1/(PEER \times RRI)$$

As you can see, these calculations can be cumbersome to do without a calculator; fortunately, Dr G Chatellier and his colleagues published the convenient nomogram shown in Figure 5.2 to help us. Alternatively, we could use the EBM calculator from our website (www.cebm.utoronto.ca).

The short way, sticking with NNT
This is a faster and easier method of estimating an NNT for our patient and is the one we usually use at the bedside or in the clinic. In this approach, the estimate we make for our patient's risk of the outcome event (if the patient were to receive just the "control" therapy) is specified relative to that of the average control patient, and expressed as a "decimal

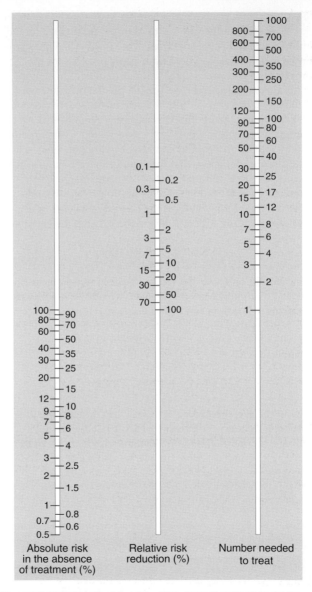

Figure 5.2 Nomogram for determining NNTs. (From Chatellier G, Zapletal E, Lemaitre D, et al. BMJ 1996; 312: 426–9.)

fraction" we call f_t. For example, if we think that our patient (if left untreated) has twice the risk of the outcome as control patients in the trial, $f_t = 2$; alternatively, if we think our patient is at only half their risk, then $f_t = 0.5$. We can use our past clinical experience and expertise in coming up with a value for f_t, or we can use any of the information sources described in the previous section. Remembering our assumption that the treatment produces a constant RRR across the range of susceptibilities, the NNT for patients just like ours is simply the reported NNT divided by f_t.

In our statin example, the study reported an NNT of 72, so we'd need to treat 72 patients like those in the trial with a statin for a mean of 5 years to prevent one more of them from experiencing a stroke.

If, however, we judge that our patient is at three times the risk of stroke without treatment as the patients in the control group, $f_t = 3$ and $NNT/f_t = 72/3 = 24$. This means that we would only need to treat 24 higher-risk patients like ours for 5 years to prevent an additional stroke.

Again, we need to consider our patient's risk of adverse events from the therapy and, to do this, we can use any of the same methods that we used to individualize our patient's NNT. Using the simplest one, we may decide that our patient is at three times the risk of adverse events as patients in the control group of the study ($f_h = 3$), or we may decide that our patient is at one-third the risk ($f_h = 0.33$). Assuming the RRI of harm is constant over the spectrum of susceptibilities, we can adjust the study NNH of 5000 with f_h (just as we did for the NNT), and generate NNH values of 1667 and 15 152 corresponding to f_h values of 3 and 0.33, respectively.

4. What are our patient's values and expectations for both the outcome we are trying to prevent and the treatment we are offering?

Thus far we've individualized the benefits and risks of therapy for our patient, but we've ignored his values and preferences. How can we incorporate these into a treatment recommendation? More importantly, how can we convert these into a form that permits our patient to make his own treatment decision? There are several models available for providing shared decision-making support, including elaborate ("Rolls Royce") ways of doing this such as a formal "clinical decision analysis" (CDA), which incorporates the patient's likelihood of the outcome events with their own values for each health state. However, performing a CDA for each patient would be too time-consuming for the busy clinician and patient, so this approach therefore usually relies on finding an existing decision analysis. To be able to use the existing decision analysis (we'll discuss this in a later section), either our patient's values (and risks) must approximate those in the analysis, or the decision analysis must provide information about the impact of variation in patient values (and risks) on the results of the decision analysis. And, even expert clinical decision analysts find them prohibitively slow to use in the real world. Clinicians can also use validated decision aids that present descriptive and probabilistic information about the target disorder, management options, and outcome events to facilitate shared decision-making. But, to date, well-validated decision aids can be tough to find. (If you're interested in finding some, take a look at Dr O'Connor's website at http://www.ohri.ca/programs/clinical_epidemiology/OPDSL/a_to_z.asp.)

Is there some quick way of incorporating patient values (say, a "Ka" version) that doesn't do too much violence to the truth? In an attempt to meet the needs of comprehensibility, applicability, and ease of use on busy clinical services, we proposed a patient-centered measure of the likelihood of being helped and harmed by an intervention based on the NNT for target events produced by the intervention (as an expression of the likelihood of being helped), the NNH for the adverse effects of therapy (to express the likelihood of being harmed), and their ratio. This result, when adjusted by an individual patient-centered conviction about the relative severities of these two events, provides an understandable, quality-adjusted, rapidly calculated measure of the "likelihood of being helped and harmed" (LHH) by a particular therapy. It goes like this:

Returning to our stroke patient and using the data in Table 5.3, we found that the ARR was 1.4% and the NNT was 72. We could use this to tell our patient that he has a 1 in 72 chance of being helped by a statin and a stroke being prevented. Similarly, looking at his risk of harm from Table 5.3, we could tell him that he has a 1 in 5000 chance of experiencing harm (e.g. rhabdomyolysis) with statin therapy. Our first approximation of his likelihood of being helped vs. harmed then becomes:

$$LHH = (1/NNT):(1/NNH)$$
$$= (1/72):(1/5000)$$
$$= 70*$$

We could then tell our patient that statin therapy is 70 times more likely to help him than to harm him. But, again, this ignores his unique risks of benefit and harm from statin therapy. We might think that his baseline risk of stroke is higher than that of patients in the control group given his age and comorbidities (and as in the previous section, we have several options for determining his PEER, but for now we'll stick with the f_t method). We could estimate f_t from our clinical experience and might decide that his risk of stroke is three times higher ($f_t = 3$) than that of the control patients (indeed, looking at a subgroup analysis in the paper, given his age, his baseline risk might be as high as 30%!); similarly, we might think his risk of rhabdomyolysis was lower than that of the control group (let's say $f_h = 0.33$). His LHH now becomes:

$$LHH = (1/NNT) \times f_t:(1/NNH) \times f_h$$
$$= (1/72) \times 3: (1/5000) \times 0.33$$
$$= 635$$

(Note that we multiply, rather than divide, by f_t in this case because we are adjusting 1/NNT.) We now tell our patient that, based on his unique risks of benefit and harm, he's

---

* Note that we could also say LHH = ARR:ARI.

635 times more likely to be helped than harmed by the therapy.

But this doesn't incorporate our patient's unique values and preferences, the consideration of which leads us to the most critical step in calculating the LHH: eliciting our patient's preferences. We ask our patient to make value judgments about the relative severity of the bad outcome we hope to prevent with therapy and the adverse event we might cause with it. We begin this in the time-honored way of describing both of them, repeating these descriptions as needed after our patient has had the chance to think about them, and discuss them with family members, etc. When the treatment option is a common one (on our service, whether to take long-term warfarin for non-valvular atrial fibrillation), we might conclude our discussion by leaving our patient with a written description of the outcomes of foregoing and accepting the treatment. An example of what information we would give a patient considering statin therapy is shown in Table 5.7. Following the review of these descriptions of the target event we hope to prevent and the adverse effects we might cause, we work with the patient to help him express how severe he considers one of them relative to the other: Is a stroke 20 times as severe as the adverse effects? Five times as severe? This can be

Table 5.7 Sample descriptions of the bad outcome we want to prevent and the potential adverse events we might cause with statin therapy

A stroke can be severe and you may have difficulty with communication, including making yourself understood (because you may have trouble getting the words out or your speech might be slurred) and understanding what others are saying to you. You may experience trouble completing your normal activities of daily living, including dressing, feeding, bathing, and toileting yourself. You will require assistance from others to complete these tasks. You have weakness of your left arm and leg and are only able to walk with use of a walker. Treatment with a medication called a "statin" can decrease the risk of stroke. You would need to take this pill daily. This treatment has side-effects, including muscle weakness and cramps. You may develop severe muscle pain and it may result in muscle breakdown; this may require admission to hospital for treatment of this condition. This side-effect is usually brief and stops once you stop taking the medication.

accomplished in a quick and simple way by asking our patient to tell us which is worse, and by how much. If the patient has difficulty making this comparison in a direct fashion, we present him with a rating scale (Figure 5.3), the ends of which are anchored at 0 (=death*) and 1 (=full health). Next, we ask our patient to place a mark where he would consider the value of the target event we hope to prevent with treatment (our patient assigned stroke a value of 0.05). Similarly, we ask him to place a second mark to correspond with his value for the adverse reactions to the treatment (our patient assigned the adverse events a value of 0.95, only a minor "disutility"). Comparing these two ratings, we can say that our patient believes that stroke is 19 (0.95/0.05) times worse than the adverse events from the therapy (we call this relative value the "severity" or "s" factor). We then ask him whether this comparison makes sense, and usually repeat this process on a second occasion to see whether this relative severity is stable.

Integrating this with our risk-adjusted LHH, the LHH becomes:

$$LHH = [(1/NNT) \times f_t \times s]{:}(1/NNH) \times f_h$$
$$= [(1/72) \times 3 \times 19]{:}(1/5000) \times 0.33$$
$$= 11\ 970$$

Thus, in the final analysis, our patient is 11 970 times more likely to be helped than harmed by statin therapy.

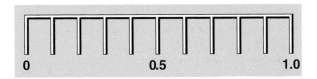

Figure 5.3 Rating scale for assessing values.

---

* Yes, our patients sometimes identify fates worse than death, in which case we extend the line below zero.

Instead of using the "s" factor, we could incorporate our patient's utilities directly into the LHH:

$$LHH = (1/NNT) \times f_t \times (1 - U_{event}):(1/NNH) \times (1 - U_{toxicity}) \times f_h$$
$$= (1/72) \times 3 \times (1 - 0.05):(1/5000 \times 0.33 \times (1 - 0.95)$$
$$= 11\ 970$$

(Note that 1 – utility provides the "disutility" associated with the outcome.)

This example can also highlight the importance of individualizing the risk of benefits and harms and incorporating our patient's values. What if our patient's risk of stroke was one-third that of patients in the control group and his risk of rhabdomyolysis was three times greater? The LHH then becomes:

$$LHH = (1/72) \times 0.33:(1/5000) \times 3$$
$$= 8$$

On reviewing his values around stroke and rhabdomyolysis, the patient decides that a stroke is four times worse than rhabdomyolysis; his LHH is therefore now 32.

If we are unsure of our patient's "f" for benefit or harm, or if our patient is uncertain about his "s" factor, we can do a sensitivity analysis by inserting other clinically sensible values for "f" and "s" and see how they affect the size and direction of the LHH.

The foregoing discussion demonstrates the "Ka" model of the LHH, but it is a far cry from the "Rolls Royce" of clinical decision analysis. We could add a few features to the basic LHH, making it into a "Jaguar" that can compare two active treatments (instead of just a placebo vs. experimental treatment as in our example). And, if there were several serious adverse events that could result from the treatment(s), we could add each of them to generate the fully adjusted LHH. Finally, as we will describe later in this chapter, we can also discount future events as in a CDA.

We've found that the LHH can be used in the busy clinical setting (median time to complete of 6.5 minutes), is intelligible to both clinicians and patients, and is unambiguously patient-centered. A version of the LHH is available on the accompanying CD; take a crack at downloading it to your PDA and let us know what you think. As other approaches in this rapidly developing field are validated in clinical settings, they will appear on our website and in future editions of this book.

Now that we've completed a critical appraisal of the paper that we retrieved, we may want to keep a permanent record of this. We find that CATs (critically appraised topics) are most useful as teaching tools. CATbanks are great practice tools if we can find sites that describe and use rigorous methodology for the creation, peer review, and updating of CATs. However, these tasks require tremendous resources, and few CATbanks that we've found meet these needs.

Further reading about individual randomized trials

Guyatt G, Rennie D, eds. Users' Guides to the Medical Literature. A Manual for Evidence-Based Clinical Practice. AMA Press: Chicago, 2002.

Sackett DL, Haynes RB, Guyatt GH, Tugwell P. Clinical Epidemiology. A Basic Science for Clinical Medicine, 2nd edn. Little, Brown: Boston, 1991.

Straus SE. Individualizing treatment decisions: the likelihood of being helped versus harmed. Eval Health Prof 2002; 25: 210–24.

A FEW WORDS ON QUALITATIVE LITERATURE

In this book, we've focused primarily on searching for and appraising quantitative literature. Qualitative research may provide us with some guidance in deciding whether we can apply the findings from quantitative studies to our patients. Qualitative research can help us to understand clinical phenomena with emphasis on understanding the experiences and values of our patients. For example, returning to our patient, we might want to look for studies that describe the experiences and feelings of patients, like him, who have taken statins, or we might want to explore literature describing why patients might not comply with statin therapy. The field of qualitative research has an extensive history in the social sciences, but its exploration and development are relatively new to clinical medicine. We don't consider ourselves experts in this area and suggest that you take a look at the references we've included at the end of this section. We've included some guides in Table 5.8 that might be useful for evaluating the validity, importance, and applicability of a qualitative study.

ARE THE RESULTS OF THIS QUALITATIVE STUDY VALID?

Table 5.8 Is the evidence from this qualitative study valid, important, and applicable?

Are the results of this qualitative study valid?

1. Was the selection of participants explicit and appropriate?
2. Were the methods for data collection and analysis explicit and appropriate?

Are the results of this valid qualitative study important?

1. Are the results impressive?

Are the valid and important results of this qualitative study applicable to my patient?

1. Do these same phenomena apply to my patient?

1. Was the selection of participants explicit and appropriate?

We'd like to find that the authors included an appropriate spectrum of patients; by appropriate we mean that they represent the population that we are interested in and who are relevant to the study question. Random sampling of participants is usually not done; instead, purposive sampling is used whereby the investigators explicitly select individuals who meet their specific criteria to reflect the experience they are assessing. For example, in a recent study evaluating the impact of the sudden acute respiratory syndrome (SARS) outbreak on professionalism amongst physicians, rather than randomly selecting a group of physicians from a list of practicing clinicians in the Province of Ontario, purposive sampling was used to ensure that both staff physicians and residents were included and that the hospitals that were affected during the outbreak were represented. The sample included participants directly involved with care of patients with SARS as well as those who were not.

2. Were the methods used for data collection and analysis explicit and appropriate?

There are many different methods for collecting and analyzing data in a qualitative study and we need to ensure that the methods are explicitly outlined. We'd suggest you refer to some of the references mentioned at the end of this section to learn more about these methods. But, there are a few questions that you can start with. Did the investigators use direct observation (or audiotapes)? Did they conduct individual face-to-face interviews or focus groups? Was a text analysis used? Did the authors develop a conceptual framework and use the collected data to challenge and refine this framework in an iterative fashion? For example, in the recent SARS study, the authors used a grounded theory approach and developed a conceptual framework using data from initial interviews. They subsequently used the data from a series of semistructured interviews to challenge this framework, and sampling of physicians continued until saturation was achieved—by this we mean no new themes were raised by the participants. The authors used investigator triangulation whereby two or more investigators analyzed the data independently. Unlike quantitative research, where we try to find articles that describe blinded outcome assessors, blinding may not always be appropriate in qualitative research because it can limit the investigator's ability to interpret the data.

ARE THE VALID RESULTS OF THIS QUALITATIVE STUDY IMPORTANT?

1. Are the results impressive?

Does the report provide sufficient detail for us to obtain a clear picture of the phenomena described? Usually the results are presented narratively, with relevant examples and quotes included to highlight themes. Sometimes authors include a quantitative component to outline dominant themes and demographic details.

ARE THE VALID, IMPORTANT RESULTS OF THIS QUALITATIVE STUDY APPLICABLE TO OUR PATIENT?
1. Do we think these same phenomena apply to our patient?
Does this paper describe patients similar to our own, and do the phenomena described seem relevant to our patient?

Further reading about qualitative studies

May N, Pope C, eds. Qualitative Research in Health Care. London: BMJ Publishing, 1996.

ADHERENCE

Given that our patient accepts a favorable LHH and embarks on treatment, everything we and the patient have invested in diagnosis, critical appraisal, and individualizing the benefits and risks of therapy comes to nothing if the patient can't or won't follow his regimen of medication taking, diet, exercise, and the like. We call this patient behavior "adherence", and stress that our use of the term carries no implications about imperialistic clinicians or submissive patients. Briefly, adherence is a major problem in health care. Usual adherence is about 50% for both short- and long-term treatments (with a range of 0–100+++%, and considerable variation within patients from week to week). The causes for low adherence rates are often not the ones we might think: age, sex, race, intelligence, and education are not important. On the other hand, long waiting times, high cost, long duration, and high complexity of treatments all lead to poor adherence. We should look for it any time a patient fails to reach a treatment goal (and especially before we increase a dose or add another drug). Irregular appointment keeping is a major clue; also, a positive response to a single question ("Have you missed one or more doses of your medication?"), when asked in a non-threatening way, generates a likelihood ratio (LR+) of 4.4

(see p. 76 for a discussion of likelihood ratios) for poor adherence (and an LR− of 0.5). If uncertainty persists, we can employ more expensive methods, such as counting pills, checking prescription databases, measuring drug levels in body fluids, and providing special pill containers that keep a time record of dosing.

Our objective in detecting low adherence is to offer our patients strategies that might help them to adhere to therapy (but before doing so we should rethink the regimen and convince ourselves that it really is worth following!). Several adherence-improving strategies have been validated in randomized trials, but none leads to huge improvements. Short-term treatment comprises exact instructions, preferably backed up by written information. Long-term measures include complex (and sometimes expensive!) combinations of greater attention and supervision: more convenient care, information on the exact regimen (but not a detailed explanation of the disease, unless the patient wants one), counseling, reminders, self-monitoring, reinforcement, and family therapy.

Further reading about adherence

Haynes RB, McDonald H, Garg AX, Montague P. Interventions to assist patients to follow prescriptions for medications. Cochrane Library Issue 3. Oxford: Update Software, 2003.

Stephenson BJ, Rowe BH, Macharia WM, Leon G, Haynes RB. Is this patient taking their medication? JAMA 1993; 269: 2779–81.

REPORTS OF SYSTEMATIC REVIEWS

It might appear that this section is out of order because the first target of any search about therapy should be a systematic review since it is the most powerful and useful evidence available. However, because the critical appraisal of a systematic review requires the skill to appraise the individual trials that comprise it, we've switched the order in this book.

A systematic review is a summary of the medical literature that uses explicit methods to systematically search, critically appraise, and synthesize the world literature on a specific issue. Its goal is to minimize both bias (usually by not only restricting itself to randomized trials, but also seeking published and unpublished reports in every language) and random error (by amassing very large numbers of individuals). Systematic reviews may, but need not, include some statistical method for combining the results of individual studies (we'll call this subset "meta-analyses"). In contrast, traditional literature reviews usually don't include an exhaustive literature search or synthesis of studies. The guides that we consider when appraising a systematic review follow. Not surprisingly, many of them (especially around importance and applicability) are the same as those for individual reports, but those for validity are different.

ARE THE RESULTS OF THIS SYSTEMATIC REVIEW VALID? (TABLE 5.9)

Table 5.9 Is the evidence from this systematic review valid?

1. Is this a systematic review of randomized trials?
2. Does it describe a comprehensive and detailed search for relevant trials?
3. Were the individual studies assessed for validity?

A less frequent point:

4. Were individual patient data (or aggregate data) used in the analysis?

1. Is this a systematic review of randomized trials?

Initially, we need to determine whether the systematic review combines randomized or non-randomized trials. We've mentioned previously in this chapter the ability of the randomized trial to reduce bias. Systematic reviews, by combining all relevant randomized trials, further reduce both bias and random error and thus provide the highest level of evidence currently achievable about the effects of health care.* In contrast, systematic reviews of non-randomized

---

* This is why the Cochrane Collaboration has been compared with the Human Genome Project; however, we think that the Cochrane Collaboration faces a greater challenge given the infinite number of trials compared with the finite number of genes!

trials can compound the problems of individually misleading trials and produce a lower quality of evidence. For this reason, if the systematic review we find includes both randomized and non-randomized trials, we avoid it unless it separates these types of trials in its analyses.

2. Does it describe a comprehensive and detailed search for relevant trials?

We need to scrutinize the methods section to determine whether it describes how the investigators found all the relevant trials. If not, we drop it and continue looking. If they did carry out a search, we seek reassurance that it went beyond standard bibliographic databases, as these have been shown to fail to label correctly up to half of the published trials in their own files. A more rigorous systematic review would include hand-searching journals (the starting point for any Cochrane Review), conference proceedings, theses, and the databanks of pharmaceutical firms, as well as contacting authors of published articles. Negative trials are less likely to be submitted and selected for publication (which could result in a false-positive conclusion in a systematic review restricted to published trials), and the other sources regularly turn up less enthusiastic unpublished trials. And if the systematic review's authors restricted their search to reports in just one language, we need to recognize that this, too, could bias the conclusions. It has been observed, for example, that bilingual German investigators were more likely to submit trials with positive results to English language journals, and those with negative results to German language journals.*

3. Were the individual studies assessed for validity?

The methods section of the report should also include a statement describing how the investigators assessed the validity of the individual studies (using criteria like those in Table 5.1). We would feel most confident in a systematic review in which multiple independent reviews of individual studies were carried out and showed good agreement.

---

* This observation applies to allopathic interventions; the situation is reversed for trials assessing complementary medical therapies!

4. Were individual patient data (or aggregate data) used for the analysis?

A less frequent point to consider is whether the authors used individual patient data (rather than summary tables or published reports) for their analysis. We'd feel more confident about the conclusions of the study, especially as it related to subgroups, if individual patient data were used, because they provide the opportunity to test promising subgroups from one trial in an identical subgroup from other trials (you might want to refer back to Table 5.6). Individual patient data also allow more reliable analyses of patients' time to specific clinical events.

IS THE VALID EVIDENCE FROM THIS SYSTEMATIC REVIEW IMPORTANT?

Once we're satisfied with the validity of the systematic review, we can turn to its results. Table 5.10 outlines the guides that we can use.

Table 5.10 Is the valid evidence from this systematic review important?
1. Are the results consistent across studies?
2. What is the magnitude of the treatment effect?
3. How precise is the treatment effect?

1. Are the results consistent across studies?

Were the effects of treatment consistent from study to study? We're more likely to believe the results of a systematic review if the results of every trial included in it show a treatment effect that is at least going in the same direction (what we'd call "qualitatively" similar results). We shouldn't expect them to show exactly the same degree of efficacy (or "quantitatively" identical results), but we should be concerned if some trials confidently conclude a beneficial effect of treatment and others in the same review powerfully exclude any benefit or demonstrate a clear-cut harm. Simply, we can look at the degree to which the confidence intervals from the various trials overlap. Ideally, we'd like to find that the investigators tested their results to see whether any lack of consistency (or "heterogeneity") was unlikely to be due to the play of chance. And, if they did find statistically significant heterogeneity, did they satisfactorily explain why it was observed (as differences in study patients, in doses of medications, in durations of therapy, outcome measurement and the like)? If study results are consistent, it is possible for the authors to use statistical methods to summarize the results; this is called "meta-analysis".

2. What is the magnitude of the treatment effect?

Just as we examined the results of single therapeutic trials, we need to find a clinically useful expression for the results of systematic reviews; here, we become victims of history and some high-level statistics (the toughest in this book). Although growing numbers of systematic reviews present their results as NNTs, most of them still use odds ratios (ORs) or relative risks (RRs).* Earlier in this chapter, we showed that the RRR doesn't preserve the CER (control event rate) or PEER (the patient's expected event rate), and this disadvantage extends to ORs and RRs. Fortunately, although ORs and RRs are of very limited use in the clinical setting, they can be converted to NNTs (or NNHs) using the formulae in Table 5.11. Better yet, we've provided the results of some typical conversions in Tables 5.12 and 5.13. And,

---

Table 5.11 Formulae to convert odds ratios (ORs) and relative risks (RRs) to NNTs

For RR <1:
$NNT = 1/(1 - RR) \times PEER$

For RR >1:
$NNT = 1/(RR - 1) \times PEER$

For OR <1:
$NNT = 1 - [PEER \times (1 - OR)]/(1 - PEER) \times (PEER) \times (1 - OR)$

For OR >1:
$NNT = 1 + [PEER \times (OR - 1)]/(1 - PEER) \times (PEER) \times (OR - 1)$

---

* The "odds ratio" is the odds of an event in a patient in the experimental group relative to that of a patient in the control group. "Relative risk" is the risk of an event in a patient in the experimental group relative to that of a patient in the control group.

Table 5.12 Translating odds ratios (ORs) to NNTs when OR <1

Patient expected event rate (PEER)	For odds ratio LESS than 1						
	0.9	0.8	0.7	0.6	0.5	0.4	0.3
0.05	209[a]	104	69	52	41	34	29[b]
0.10	110	54	36	27	21	18	15
0.20	61	30	20	14	11	10	8
0.30	46	22	14	10	8	7	5
0.40	40	19	12	9	7	6	4
0.50	38	18	11	8	6	5	4
0.70	44	20	13	9	6	5	4
0.90	101[c]	46	27	18	12	9	4[d]

[a] The relative risk reduction (RRR) here is 10%.
[b] The RRR here is 49%.
[c] The RRR here is 1%.
[d] The RRR here is 9%.
Adapted from John Geddes (personal communication, 1999).

Table 5.13 Translating odds ratios (ORs) to NNTs when OR >1

Patient expected event rate (PEER)	For odds ratio GREATER than 1						
	1.1	1.25	1.5	1.75	2	2.25	2.5
0.05	212	86	44	30	23	18	16
0.10	113	46	24	16	13	10	9
0.20	64	27	14	10	8	7	6
0.30	50	21	11	8	7	6	5
0.40	44	19	10	8	6	5	5
0.50	42	18	10	8	6	6	5
0.70	51	23	13	10	9	8	7
0.90	121	55	33	25	22	19	18

The numbers in the body of the table are the NNTs for the corresponding ORs at that particular PEER. This table applies both when a good outcome is increased by therapy, and when a side-effect is caused by therapy.
Adapted from John Geddes (personal communication, 1999).

finally, we can take a short-cut and use the EBM calculator on our website and CD which allows us to convert an OR to an NNT at the click of a button (www.cebm.utoronto.ca). We interpret the NNTs and NNHs derived from systematic reviews in the same way as we would for individual trials.

ARE THE VALID, IMPORTANT RESULTS OF THIS SYSTEMATIC REVIEW APPLICABLE TO OUR PATIENT? (TABLE 5.14)

> **Table 5.14** Is this valid and important evidence from a systematic review applicable to our patient?
>
> 1. Is our patient so different from those in the study that its results cannot apply?
> 2. Is the treatment feasible in our setting?
> 3. What are our patient's potential benefits and harms from the therapy?
> 4. What are our patient's values and expectations for both the outcome we are trying to prevent and the adverse effects we may cause?

A systematic review provides an overall, average effect of therapy, which may be derived from a quite heterogeneous population. How do we apply this evidence to our individual patient? The same way we did it for individual trials, by applying the guides for applicability listed in Table 5.14. One advantage that systematic reviews have over most randomized trials is that the former may provide precise information on subgroups, which can help us to individualize the evidence to our own patients. In order to do this, however, we need to remind ourselves of the cautions about subgroups we've summarized in Table 5.6.

Further reading about systematic reviews

Egger M, Altman DG, Smith GD. Systematic Reviews in Health Care. London: BMJ Books, 2001.

Glasziou P, Irwig L, Bain C, Colditz G. Systematic reviews in health care: a practical guide. Cambridge: Cambridge University Press, 2001.

Guyatt G, Rennie D, eds. Users' Guides to the Medical Literature. A Manual for Evidence-Based Clinical Practice. Chicago: AMA Press, 2002.

PRACTICING EBM IN REAL-TIME
Using pre-appraised evidence

Often, tracking down and appraising the primary literature takes time that we can't afford during clinical practice; instead we can try to find high-quality pre-appraised evidence (as described in Ch. 2). For example, we could look for an answer to our question about statin use in *Clinical Evidence*. (As mentioned in Chapter 2, *Clinical Evidence* uses explicit, rigorous methods to retrieve, appraise, summarize, and update relevant evidence.) In less than 30 seconds we are able to find a relevant section in *Clinical Evidence* describing the evidence for cholesterol reduction in patients with prior TIA (transient ischemic attack). It mentions that a systematic review and one additional RCT looked at the effects on CAD and stroke of reducing cholesterol with a statin; the RCTs didn't specifically aim to include people with prior TIA, but a subsequent RCT did so. The resource highlights the benefits and harms of statin therapy and the CER, EER, and OR are provided. Using this pre-appraised evidence, we can obtain the answer to our clinical question in less than 30 seconds, making it feasible to practice EBM in real-time at the bedside! Take a look at the *Clinical Evidence* website (www.clinicalevidence.org); access to this resource can be arranged for a limited time so that you can try this search yourself.

REPORTS OF CLINICAL DECISION ANALYSES

Occasionally, when we are attempting to answer a question about therapy, the results of our search will yield a clinical decision analysis (CDA). A CDA applies explicit, quantitative methods to compare the likely consequences of pursuing different treatment strategies, and integrates the risks of benefit and harm associated with the various treatment options with values associated with the treatments and with potential outcomes. A CDA starts with a diagram called a "decision tree"; this illustrates the target disorder, the alternative treatment strategies, and their possible outcomes. An example of a simple decision tree is shown in Figure 5.4;

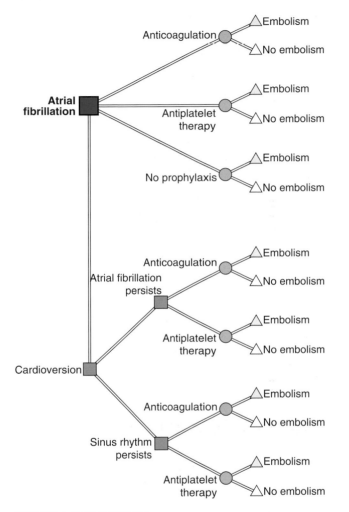

Figure 5.4 A simple decision tree.

this looks at the possible strategies for the management of atrial fibrillation, including anticoagulation, antiplatelet therapy, no antithrombotic prophylaxis, and cardioversion. The point at which a treatment decision is made is marked with a square box. The possible outcomes that arise from the treatment strategies follow this decision node and are preceded by circles (called "chance nodes"). The probabilities for each of these events are estimated from the literature (hopefully with a modicum of accuracy!), or occasionally from the clinician's clinical expertise. Triangles are placed at the end of each outcome branch, and the patient's "utility" for each outcome is placed here. A "utility" is the measure of a person's preference for a health state, and is usually expressed as a decimal from 0 to 1. Typically, perfect health is assigned a value of 1, and death is assigned a value of 0; however, there are some outcomes that patients may think are worse than death, so the scale may need to be extended below zero. Formal methods should be used to elicit utilities, including the standard gamble and time trade-off techniques. Sometimes CDAs may use life-years, quality-adjusted life-years (QALYs, where a year in a higher-quality health state contributes more to the outcome than a year in a poor-quality health state), or cases of disease or complications that are prevented. The utility of each outcome is multiplied by the probability that it will occur; this is summed for each chance node in the treatment branch to generate an average utility for that branch of the tree. The "winning" strategy, and preferred course of clinical action, is the one that leads to the highest utility. Note that this figure outlines a very simple tree, although we could make it fancy and include the possibility of patients experiencing more than one outcome or health state.

While on clinical services, we've encountered an insurmountable time barrier to the use of CDAs (and as mentioned, in discussions with our colleagues with significant expertise in this area, few are able to tackle them in real-time). To be done right, they have to generate and integrate probabilities and patient utilities for all pertinent outcomes, and particularize these probabilities and utilities to a specific patient. The result is elegant, and we sometimes wish we could do it for all our patients, but the process takes us an average of 3 days to complete just one simple tree. We've opted to use the more rough-and-ready but humanly feasible approaches for integrating evidence and patients' values such as the LHH. We don't consider ourselves experts at CDA; if you are interested in reading more about how to do them, check out the references at the end of this section.

But even if we don't do CDAs, we sometimes read reports of them, and the rest of this section will briefly describe how we decide whether they are valid, important, and applicable to a patient. The guides that we use to do this follow.

ARE THE RESULTS OF THIS CDA VALID? (TABLE 5.15)

Table 5.15 Is this evidence from a CDA valid?
1. Were all important therapeutic alternatives (including no treatment) and outcomes included?
2. Are the probabilities of the outcomes valid and credible?
3. Are the utilities of the outcomes valid and credible?

The CDA should include all the treatment strategies and the full range of outcomes (both good and bad) that we think are important. For example, if we are interested in looking at a CDA that might help us determine the best management of patients with non-valvular atrial fibrillation and the CDA we find doesn't include aspirin as an alternative treatment to anticoagulants, we should be skeptical about its usefulness (since both work, albeit to different degrees). A CDA should explicitly describe a comprehensive systematic process that was used to identify, select, and combine the best external evidence into probabilities for all the important clinical outcomes. There may be some uncertainty around a probability estimate, and the authors should specify a range; this may come from the range of values from different studies, or from a 95% confidence interval from a single study or systematic review. The methods that were used to assess the evidence for validity (see p. 117) should also be included in the study.

If a systematic review was not found to provide an estimate of the probability, were the results of the studies that were found combined in some sensible way? Finally, some investigators may use expert opinion to generate probability estimates, if these aren't available in the clinical literature, but these estimates won't be as valid as those obtained from evidence-based sources.

Were the utilities obtained in an explicit and sensible way from valid sources? Ideally, utilities are measured in patients using valid, standardized methods such as the standard gamble or time trade-off techniques. Occasionally, investigators will use values already present in the clinical literature or values obtained by "consensus opinion" from experts. These latter two methods are not nearly as credible as measuring utilities directly in appropriate patients.

Ideally, in a high-quality CDA, the investigators should "discount" future events. For example, most people wouldn't trade a year of perfect health now for one 20 years in the future—we usually value the present greater than the future. Discounting the utility will take this into account.

If we think the CDA has satisfied all of the above criteria, we move on to considering whether the results of this CDA are important. If it doesn't satisfy the criteria, we'll have to go back to our search.

ARE THE VALID RESULTS OF THIS CDA IMPORTANT? (TABLE 5.16)

Table 5.16 Is this valid evidence from a CDA important?
1. Did one course of action lead to clinically important gains?
2. Was the same course of action preferred despite clinically sensible changes in probabilities and utilities?

Was there a clear "winner" in this CDA, so that one course of action clearly led to a higher average utility? Surprisingly, experts in this area often conclude that average gains in QALYs of as little as 2 months are worth pursuing (especially when their confidence intervals are big, so that some patients enjoy really big gains in QALYs). On the other hand, gains of a few days to a few weeks are usually considered "toss-ups" in which both courses of action lead to identical outcomes and there is nothing to choose between them.

Before accepting the results of a positive CDA, we need to make sure it determined whether clinically sensible changes in probabilities or utilities altered its conclusion. If this "sensitivity analysis" generated no switch in the designation of the preferred treatment, it is a robust analysis. If, on the other hand, the designation of the preferred treatment is sensitive to small changes in one or more probabilities or utilities, the results of the CDA are uncertain and it may not provide any important guidance for our patient and us.

ARE THE VALID, IMPORTANT RESULTS OF THIS CDA APPLICABLE TO OUR PATIENT? (TABLE 5.17)

Table 5.17 Is this valid and important evidence from a CDA applicable to our patient?

1. Do the probabilities in this CDA apply to our patient?
2. Can our patient state his/her utilities in a stable, usable form?

Once we've decided that the conclusions of a CDA are both valid and important, we still need to decide whether we can apply it to our patient. Are our patient's probabilities of the various outcomes included in the sensitivity analysis? If they lie outside the range tested, we'll need to either recalculate it or at least be very cautious in following its recommendations. Similarly, we might want to generate utilities for our patient to see if they fall within the range tested in the CDA. A crude technique that we use on our clinical service begins by drawing a line on a sheet of paper with two anchor points on it: one at the top labeled "perfect health" which is given a value of 1, and one near the bottom labeled "death" which is given a score of 0 (making the line precisely 10 or 20 cm long helps, as you'll see). After explaining it, we ask the patient to mark the places on the scale that correspond to his current state of health and to all the other outcomes that might result from the choice of interventions. The locations that the patient selects are used to represent the utilities (if time permits, we leave the scale with the patient so that he can reflect on, and perhaps revise, the utilities). We can then see whether our patient's utilities (both initially and on reflection) lie within the boundaries of the study's sensitivity analysis.

FURTHER READING ABOUT CLINICAL DECISION ANALYSIS

Guyatt G, Rennie D, eds. Users' Guides to the Medical Literature. A Manual for Evidence-Based Clinical Practice. Chicago: AMA Press, 2002.

Hunink M, Glasziou P, Siegel J, Weeks J, Pliskin J, Elstein A, Weinstein M. Decision Making in Health and Medicine: Integrating Evidence and Values. Cambridge: Cambridge University Press, 2001.

REPORTS OF ECONOMIC ANALYSES

Sometimes our search for an answer to a therapeutic or other clinical question will yield an economic analysis that compares the costs and consequences of different management decisions. We warn you at the outset that economic analyses are difficult to interpret and often controversial (even among health economists!), and we won't pretend to describe all their nuances here (if you are interested in understanding them, we've suggested some additional resources at the end of this section). Economic analyses are very demanding for their investigators, and for us readers as well. For example, they teach us to stop thinking about the costs of a new treatment in terms of pounds and pence/dollars and cents, and to start thinking about them in terms of the other things we can't do if we use our scarce resources to fund this new treatment. This "cost as sacrifice" is better known as "opportunity cost" and is a useful way of thinking in everyday practice; for example, when we internists "borrow" a bed from our surgical colleagues in order to admit a medical emergency tonight, the opportunity cost of our decision includes canceling tomorrow's elective surgery on the patient for whom the bed was reserved.

These papers are pretty tough to read and you might want to confine your initial searches to the evidence-based journals (such as *ACP Journal Club, Evidence Based Medicine*, and the like), which not only provide a standard, clear format for reporting economic analyses but also provide expert commentaries. The following guides should help you decide whether an economic analysis is valid, important, and useful.

ARE THE RESULTS OF THIS ECONOMIC ANALYSIS VALID? (TABLE 5.18)

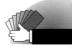

Table 5.18 Is this evidence from an economic analysis valid?
1. Are all well-defined courses of action compared?
2. Does it provide a specified view from which the costs and consequences are being viewed?
3. Does it cite comprehensive evidence on the efficacy of alternatives?
4. Does it identify all the costs and consequences we think it should and select credible and accurate measures of them?
5. Was the type of analysis appropriate for the question posed?

We need to begin by remembering that economic analyses are about choices and must therefore ensure that the study included all the sensible, alternative courses of action (e.g. anticoagulation, antiplatelet therapy, and cardioversion for patients with non-valvular atrial fibrillation) rather than just one or two of them. If, for example, we found a report that only described the costs of antiplatelet therapy for patients with non-valvular atrial fibrillation, that's an exercise in accounting, not economic analysis, and it wouldn't help us. A valid economic analysis also has to specify the point of view from which the costs and outcomes are being viewed. Did the authors specify if costs and consequences are evaluated from the perspective of the patient, hospital or local government? For example, a hospital might shy away from inpatient cardioversion in favor of discharging a patient with non-valvular atrial fibrillation on anticoagulants that would be paid for from the family physician's drug budget, whereas society as a whole would want the most cost-effective approach from an overall point of view.

Because economic analyses assume (rather than prove) that the alternative courses of action have highly predictable effects, we need to determine whether they cite and summarize solid evidence on the efficacy of alternatives (the same caution we must remember when reading a CDA). So, was an explicit and sensible process used to identify and appraise the evidence that would satisfy the criteria for validity displayed back in Table 5.1?

All the costs and effects of the treatment should be identified, and credible measures should have been made of all of them. The cost side here can be tricky, since we may want the report to include all the costs, including direct costs (e.g. cost of medication, hospitalization) and indirect costs (e.g. time lost from work). Moreover, a high-quality economic analysis should also include (and explain!) discounting future costs and outcomes (to acknowledge the fact that a bird in the hand is worth two in next year's bush).

We need to consider if the type of analysis was appropriate for the question the investigators posed, and this isn't as hard as it sounds. If the question was "Is there a cheaper (but equally effective) way to care for this patient?", the paper should ignore the outcomes and simply compare costs (a "cost minimization" analysis). If the question was "Which way of treating this patient gives the greatest health `bang for the buck'?", the method of analysis is determined by the sorts of outcomes being compared. If outcomes are identical for all the treatment alternatives (say, whether it's cheaper to prevent embolic stroke in non-ventricular atrial fibrillation patients with aspirin or warfarin), the appropriate analysis is a "cost-effectiveness" analysis. If, however, the outcomes as well as the interventions differ (Do we get a bigger bang for our buck treating kids for leukemia or the elderly for Alzheimer's dementia?), the authors will have had to come up with some way of measuring these disparate outcomes with the same yardstick, and there are two of these. They could convert all outcomes into monetary values: a "cost–benefit" analysis. The challenge in cost–benefit analysis is setting monetary values: Should they be earning power (in which case we treat the kids and warehouse the elderly), or can we put a value on life itself? No wonder that cost–benefit analysis lacks popularity. The other common yardstick for disparate outcomes is their social (rather than monetary) value: How do patients view their desirability compared with other outcomes (including perfect health and death, and fates worse than death)? A shorthand economic term for these preferences is "utility"; utilities can be combined with time to generate QALYs (e.g. 1 year in perfect health is judged equivalent to 3 years in a post-stroke state whose utility is only 0.3). The corresponding economic analysis is called "cost–utility" analysis.

If the economic analysis fails the above tests for validity, it's back to searching. If it passes, we can proceed to considering whether its valid results are important.

ARE THE VALID RESULTS OF THIS ECONOMIC ANALYSIS IMPORTANT? (TABLE 5.19)

Table 5.19 Is this valid evidence from an economic analysis important?
1. Are the resulting costs, or cost per unit of health gained, clinically significant?
2. Did the results of this economic analysis change with sensible changes to costs and effectiveness?

Specifically, are the resulting costs, or cost per unit of health gained, clinically significant? We need to consider whether the intervention will provide a benefit at an acceptable cost. If it is a "cost-minimization" analysis, we should consider if the difference in cost is big enough to warrant switching to a cheaper one. For a cost-effectiveness analysis, is the difference in effectiveness great enough for us to want to spend the difference? If a cost–utility analysis was done, how do the QALYs generated from spending resources on this treatment compare with those that would result if we spent them in other ways? This comparison is made superficially easier by the growing popularity of cost–utility "league tables".*

ARE THE VALID, IMPORTANT RESULTS OF THIS ECONOMIC ANALYSIS APPLICABLE TO OUR PATIENT/PRACTICE? (TABLE 5.20)

Table 5.20 Is this valid and important evidence from an economic analysis applicable to our patient?

1. Do the costs in the economic analysis apply in our setting?
2. Are the treatments likely to be effective in our setting?

As usual, we begin by considering whether our patient is so different from those included in the study that its results are not applicable. We can do this by estimating our patient's probabilities of the various outcomes, and by asking the patient to generate the utilities for these outcomes. If these values fall within the ranges used in the analysis, we can be satisfied that the "effectiveness" results can be applied to our patient. Next we can consider whether the intervention would be used in the same way in our practice. We compare the costs of applying this intervention in the study and carrying it out in our own setting. Costs may be different because of different practice patterns and because local prices for resources vary. If we think they would be different, are our personal cost estimates in the range tested in the sensitivity analysis?

If the paper satisfies all of the above tests, we can celebrate. But if it fails any of them, it's back to the searching process!

---

* If you want to learn more about league tables, we'd suggest you take a look at: Mason J, Drummond M, Torrance G. Some guidelines on the use of cost-effectiveness league tables. BMJ 1993; 306: 570–2.

Further reading about economic analysis

Guyatt G, Rennie D, eds. Users' Guides to the Medical Literature. A Manual for Evidence-Based Clinical Practice. Chicago: AMA Press, 2002.

REPORTS OF CLINICAL PRACTICE GUIDELINES

It seems that we cannot scan a journal or open our mail without finding information about a new clinical practice guideline. Clinical practice guidelines are systematically developed statements to help clinicians and patients with decisions about appropriate health care for specific clinical circumstances.[8] Huge amounts of time and money are being invested in their production, application, and dissemination. Unfortunately, this often occurs with unnecessary duplication; we recently completed a search for guidelines on the management of heart failure and we were daunted when we retrieved over 1000 citations! This next section is to help busy clinicians to decide whether a guideline is worth using.

In a nutshell, if we're considering using a guideline, we should think of it as having two distinct components, as depicted in Table 5.21: first, the evidence summary ("here's the average effect of this intervention on the typical patient who accepts it"); second, the detailed instructions for applying that evidence to our patient. Then we should look at the two components individually. We apply our eye and nose to the first component, the evidence summary: our eye, to see if all the relevant evidence has been tracked down and graded for its validity; and our nose, to smell whether it has updated its review recently enough to still be fresh. Then we apply our ear to the second component to listen for any "killer Bs" (Burden, Beliefs, Bargain, Barriers; Table 5.22) in our neighborhood that would make its detailed instructions impossible to execute. And if we're asked to (help) write one, we should never volunteer to labor in the first component (except as a member of a Cochrane Review Group), but insist that we be appointed to the second component as the local "B-keeper".

Table 5.21 The two components of practice guidelines

	Evidence component	Detailed instructional component
Bottom line	"Here's the typical effect of this diagnostic/ therapeutic/ preventive intervention on the typical patient."	"Here is exactly what to do to/with this patient."
Underlying requirements	Validity, importance, up-to-datedness	Local relevance
Expertise required by those executing this component	Human biology, consumerism, clinical epidemiology, biostatistics, database searching	Clinical practice, patient values, current practice, local geography, local economics, local sociology, local politics, local traditions
Site where this component should be performed	National or international	Local
Form of output	Levels of evidence	Grades of recommendations, detailed instructions, flowcharts, protocols

Valid guidelines create their evidence components from systematic reviews of all the relevant worldwide literature. The reviews that provide the evidence components for guidelines are "necessity-driven", and synthesize the best evidence (even if it is of shaky quality) that can be found to guide an urgent decision that has to be made. It necessarily follows that some recommendations in the second component of a guideline may be derived from evidence of high validity and others from evidence that is much more liable to error.

ARE THE RESULTS OF THIS PRACTICE GUIDELINE VALID?
Detailed guides for assessing the validity of practice guidelines have been developed using rigorous methodology, and we'd suggest that you turn to these if you are

Table 5.22 The killer Bs
1. Is the **B**urden of illness (frequency in our community, or our patient's pre-test probability or expected event rate, PEER) too low to warrant implementation?
2. Are the **B**eliefs of individual patients or communities about the value of the interventions or their consequences incompatible with the guideline?
3. Would the opportunity cost of implementing this guideline constitute a bad **B**argain in the use of our energy or our community's resources?
4. Are the **B**arriers (geographic, organizational, traditional, authoritarian, legal, or behavioral) so high that it is not worth trying to overcome them?

particularly interested in this topic (www.agreecollaborative.org). In this section, we present a more basic version that you can use when appraising the validity of guidelines (Table 5.23).

Similar to high-quality CDAs and economic analyses, valid practice guidelines should include all relevant strategies (e.g. for diagnosis, screening, prognosis, and/or treatment), and the full range of outcomes (including the good and the bad) that are important. For example, a recent guideline by the Canadian Task Force for Preventive Health Care found that there was fair evidence of no benefit and good evidence of harm with routine teaching of self-breast examinations in women aged 40–69 years.[9] It was crucial for this guideline to include data not only on the impact of this screening intervention on mortality, but also on the potential harm, including the emotional distress associated with unnecessary breast biopsies.

Table 5.23 Guides for deciding whether a guideline is valid
1. Did its developers carry out a comprehensive, reproducible literature review within the past 12 months?
2. Is each of its recommendations both tagged by the level of evidence upon which it is based and linked to a specific citation?

A valid practice guideline should also include a comprehensive, reproducible literature review. A comprehensive review needs to include all relevant articles in all relevant languages (for example, some of the most important evidence for guidelines about family supports for patients with schizophrenia was published in Mandarin). Ideally, the guideline should describe explicitly the methods used to retrieve, appraise, and synthesize the evidence.

Although we'd like to see therapy recommendations supported by evidence from systematic reviews of randomized trials, as we've discussed previously such evidence might not always be available. It follows, therefore, that some guideline recommendations may be derived from high-quality evidence and others from evidence that is more prone to error. Because strength of evidence supporting guideline recommendations may vary, it is useful to have the strength of recommendations graded on the quality of evidence found. Accordingly, it is important that these different "levels" of evidence are acknowledged in tying the evidence to the clinical recommendations. Only in this way can we separate the really solid recommendations from the tenuous ones, and (if we want to appraise the evidence for ourselves) track them back to their sources. This need was recognized back in the 1970s by the Canadian Task Force on the Periodic Health Exam,[10] and ever more sophisticated ways of describing and categorizing levels of evidence have followed.[11] In the present era, they have been an important element of at least some of the clinical texts on "evidence-based practice" in which each clinical recommendation is accompanied by an icon denoting the level of evidence that was employed in generating it. Table 5.24 has some examples of levels of evidence for therapy studies that we've found useful.

As you can see, satisfying these validity guides is a formidable task, and successful development of guidelines requires a combination of clinical, informational, and methodological skills, plus lots of time and money. For this reason, this first component of guideline development is best filled by a national or international collaboration of sufficient

Table 5.24 Levels of evidence for therapy studies

Level of evidence	Therapy/prevention/etiology/harm
1a	Systematic review with homogeneity of RCTs[a]
1b	Individual RCT with narrow confidence interval[b]
1c	All or none[c]
2a	Systematic review (with homogeneity) of cohort studies
2b	Individual cohort study (including low-quality RCT; e.g. <80% follow-up)
3a	Systematic review (with homogeneity) of case–control study
3b	Individual case–control study
4	Case series (and poor quality cohort and case–control studies)[d]
5	Expert opinion without explicit critical appraisal, or based on physiology, bench research or "first principles"

[a] By homogeneity we mean that a systematic review is free of worrisome variations (heterogeneity) in the directions and degrees of results between individual studies. Not all systematic reviews with statistically significant heterogeneity are worrisome, and not all worrisome heterogeneity need be statistically significant.

[b] For example, if the confidence interval excludes a clinically important benefit or harm.

[c] Met when all patients died before the treatment became available, but some now survive on it; or when some patients died before the treatment became available, but now none die on it.

[d] By poor-quality cohort study, we mean one that failed to clearly define comparison groups and/or failed to measure exposures and outcomes in the same (preferably blinded) objective way in both exposed and non-exposed individuals, and/or failed to identify or appropriately control known confounders, and/or failed to carry out a sufficiently long and complete follow-up of patients. By poor-quality case–control study, we mean one that failed to clearly define comparison groups, and/or failed to measure exposures and outcomes in the same blinded, objective way in both cases and controls, and/or failed to identify or appropriately control known cofounders.

scope and size to not only carry out the systematic review but to update it as often as important new evidence appears on the scene.

IS THIS VALID GUIDELINE APPLICABLE TO MY PATIENT/PRACTICE/HOSPITAL/COMMUNITY?

The first (and most important) advice here is that, if a guideline developed out of town tells us how to treat our patients in town, we should be very wary about its applicability. Good guideline development clearly separates the evidence component ("here's what you can expect to achieve in the typical patient who accepts this intervention") from the detailed recommendations component ("admit to an intensive care unit (ICU), carry out this ELISA test, order that treatment, monitor it minute by minute, and have your neurosurgeon examine the patient twice a day"). What if we have no ICU, can't afford ELISA tests, have to get special Ministry of Health permission to use the treatment, are caring for a patient whose next of kin doesn't like this sort of treatment, are chronically short-staffed, and our nearest neurosurgeon is 3 hours away?

The applicability of a guideline depends on the extent to which it is in harmony or conflict with four local (sometimes patient-specific) factors; these are summarized as the potential "killer Bs" of Table 5.22. If you hear any of these four bees buzzing in your ear when you consider the applicability of a guideline, be cautious.

First, is the "burden" of illness too low to warrant implementation? Is the target disorder rare in our area (e.g. malaria in northern Canada)? Or is the outcome we hope to detect or prevent unlikely in our patient (e.g. the pre-test probability for significant coronary stenosis in a young woman with non-anginal chest pain)? If so, implementing the guideline may not only be a waste of time and money, but it might also do more harm than good. Reflecting on this "B" requires that we consider our patient's risk of the event and their unique circumstances as we do when assessing the applicability of any piece of evidence (Table 5.5).

Second, are our patients' or community's "beliefs" about the values or utilities of the interventions themselves, or the benefits and harms they produce, compatible with the guideline's recommendations? Ideally, guidelines should include some mention of values, who assigned these values (are they patient-derived or author-derived?), and whether they came from one source or many sources. The values assumed in a guideline, either explicitly or implicitly, may not match those in our patient or our community. Even if the values seem, on average, to be reasonable, we must avoid forcing them on individual patients because patients with identical risks may not have the same beliefs, values, and preferences as those who are used or assumed in the guideline, and some may be quite averse to undergoing the recommended procedures. For example, early breast cancer patients with identical risks, given the same information about chemotherapy, make fundamentally different treatment decisions based on how they weigh the long-term benefit of reducing the risk of recurrence against the short-term harm of being nauseated and losing their hair.[12] Similarly, patients with severe angina at identical risk of coronary events, given the same information about treatment options, exhibit sharply contrasting treatment preferences because of the different values they place on the risks and benefits of surgery.[13] Although the average beliefs in a community are appropriate for deciding, for example, whether chemotherapy or surgery should be paid for with public funds, decisions for individual patients must reflect their own personal beliefs and preferences.

Third, would the opportunity cost of implementing this guideline—rather than some other one(s)—constitute a "bargain" in the use of our energy or our community's resources? We need to remember that the cost of shortening the waiting list for surgery is lengthening that for family therapy. As decision-making of this sort gets decentralized, different communities are bound to make different economic decisions, and "health care by postal code" will and ought to occur, especially under democratic governments.

And finally, are there insurmountable "barriers" to implementing the guideline in our patient (whose preferences indicate they'd be more likely to be harmed than helped by the intervention/investigation, or who would flatly refuse the investigations or intervention), or in our community? Barriers can be geographic (if the required interventions are not available locally), organizational (one of us visited a hospital where the emergency department is located at one site and the neurologists who initiate use of urgent thrombolysis in stroke patients are located at a second hospital, more than 30 minutes away), traditional ("But we've always done it the other way!"), authoritarian ("But you've always done it my way!"), legal (fear of litigation if a usual but useless practice is abandoned), or behavioral (when clinicians fail to apply the guideline or patients fail to take their medicine). If there are major barriers, the potential benefits of implementing a guideline may not be worth the effort and resources (or opportunity costs) required to overcome them.

Changing our own, our colleagues', and our patients' behavior often requires much more than simply knowing what to do. If implementing a guideline requires changing behavior, we need to identify which barriers are operating and what we can do about them. Significant attention is now being paid to evaluate methods of overcoming these barriers, including changing physician behavior. Indeed, the finding that providing evidence from clinical research is a necessary but not sufficient condition for the provision of optimal care has created interest in knowledge translation, the scientific study of the methods for closing the knowledge-to-practice gap, and the analysis of barriers and facilitators inherent in the process.[14]

So, in deciding whether a valid guideline is applicable to our patient/practice/hospital/community, we need to identify the four "Bs" that pertain to the guideline and decide whether they can be reconciled with its application (or whether we are facing one or more "killer Bs"). Note that none of these "Bs" (even when present as "killer Bs") has any effect on the validity of the evidence component of the guideline. Note also that the only people who are "experts" in the "Bs" are the patients and providers at the sharp edge of implementing the application component.

n-OF-1 TRIALS

You may not always be able to find a randomized trial or systematic review relevant to your patient. Traditionally, when faced with this dilemma, we clinicians have conducted a "trial of therapy", during which we start our patient on a treatment and follow him to determine whether the symptoms improve or worsen while on treatment. Performing this standard trial of therapy may be misleading (and is prone to bias) for several reasons:

1. Some target disorders are self-limited and patients may get better on their own.

2. Both extreme lab values and clinical signs, if left untreated and reassessed later, often return to normal.

3. A placebo can lead to substantial improvement in symptoms.

4. Both our own and our patient's expectations about the success or failure of a treatment can bias conclusions about whether a treatment actually works.

5. Polite patients may exaggerate the effects of therapy.

If a treatment was used during any of the above situations, it would tend to appear efficacious when in fact it was useless.

The n-of-1 trial applies the principles of rigorous clinical trial methodology to overcome these problems when trying to determine the best treatment for an individual patient. It randomizes time, and assigns the patient (using concealed randomization and hopefully blinding of the patient and clinician) active therapy or placebo at different times, so that the patient undergoes cycles of experimental and control treatment, resulting in multiple crossovers to help both our patient and us to decide on the best therapy. It is employed when there is significant doubt about whether a treatment might be helpful in a particular patient, and is most successful when directed toward the control of symptoms or relapses resulting from a chronic disease.

Guides that we use in deciding whether or not to execute an n-of-1 trial are listed in Table 5.25. The crucial first step in this process is to have a discussion with the patient to determine his interest, willingness to participate, expectations of the treatment, and desired outcomes. Next

Table 5.25 Guides for n-of-1 randomized trials

1. Is an n-of-1 trial indicated for our patient?
   - Is the effectiveness of the treatment really in doubt for our patient?
   - Will the treatment, if effective, be continued long-term?
   - Is our patient willing and eager to collaborate in designing and carrying out an n-of-1 trial?

2. Is an n-of-1 trial feasible in our patient?
   - Does the treatment have a rapid onset?
   - Does the treatment cease to act soon after it is discontinued?
   - Is the optimal treatment duration feasible?
   - Can outcomes that are relevant and important to our patient be measured?
   - Can we establish sensible criteria for stopping the trial?
   - Can an unblinded run-in period be conducted?

3. Is an n-of-1 trial feasible in our practice setting?
   - Is there a pharmacist available to help?
   - Are strategies for interpreting the trial data in place?

4. Is the n-of-1 study ethical?
   - Is approval by our medical research ethics committee necessary?

we need to determine if formal ethics approval is required.* If, after reviewing these guides, it is decided to do an n-of-1 trial, we use the following tactics (they are described in detail elsewhere):†

1. Come to agreement with our patient on the symptoms, signs, or other manifestations of his target disorder that we want to improve, and set up a data collection method so that the data can be recorded regularly.

2. Determine (in collaboration with a pharmacist and our patient) the active and comparison (usually placebo) treatments, treatment durations, and rules for stopping a treatment period.

3. Set up pairs of treatment periods in which our patient receives the experimental therapy during one period and the placebo during the other (with the order of treatment randomized).

---

* At our institutions this is variable; in some places ethics and written consent are required and at others not, because the objective is improved care for an individual patient, who is our co-investigator.

† Guyatt G, Rennie D. Users' Guides to the Medical Literature. Chicago: AMA Press, 2002.

4. If possible, both we and our patient remain blind to the treatment being given during any period, even when we examine the results at the end of the pair of periods.

5. Pairs of treatment periods are continued and analyzed until we decide to unblind the results and decide whether to continue the active therapy or abandon it.

Further reading about n-of-1 trials

Guyatt GH, Keller JL, Jaeschke R, Rosenbloom D, Adachi JD, Newhouse MT. The n-of-1 randomized controlled trial: clinical usefulness. Our three-year experience. Ann Intern Med 1990; 112: 293–9.

Guyatt G, Sackett D, Adachi J, Roberts R, Chong J, Rosenbloom D, Keller JA. A clinician's guide for conducting randomized trials in individual patients. CMAJ 1998; 139: 497–503.

Sackett DL, Haynes RB, Guyatt GH, Tugwell P. Clinical Epidemiology: A Basic Science for Clinical Medicine, 2nd edn. Boston: Little, Brown, 1991.

REFERENCES

1 MRC/BHF. Heart Protection Study. Lancet 2002; 360: 7–22.

2 Stampfer MJ, Colditz GA. Estrogen replacement therapy and coronary heart disease: a quantitative assessment of the epidemiologic evidence. Prev Med 1991; 20: 47–63.

3 Hulley S, Grady D, Bush T, et al. Randomized trial of estrogen plus progestin for secondary prevention of coronary heart disease in postmenopausal women. JAMA 1998; 280: 605–13.

4 Rossouw JE, Anderson G, Prentice RL, et al. Risks and benefits of estrogen and progestin in healthy postmenopausal women: principal results from the Women's Health Initiative randomized controlled trial. JAMA 2002; 288: 321–3.

5 Barnett HJ, Taylor DW, Eliaszew M, et al. Benefits of carotid endarterectomy in patients with symptomatic moderate or severe stenosis. N Engl J Med 1998; 339: 1415–25.

6 Devereaux PJ, Manns B, Ghali WH, et al. Physician interpretations and textbook definitions of blinding terminology in randomized control trials. JAMA 2001; 285: 2000–3.

7 ACP Journal Club 2003; 138: 2.

8 Institute of Medicine. Clinical Practice Guidelines: Directions for a New Program. Washington, DC: National Academy Press, 1990.

9 Canadian Task Force for Preventive Health Care. Preventive health care, 2001 update: Should women be routinely taught breast self-examination to screen for breast cancer? CMAJ 2001; 164: 134.

10 The Canadian Task Force on the Periodic Health Examination. The periodic health examination. CMAJ 1979; 121: 1093–254.

11 Guyatt G, Rennie D, eds. Users' Guides to the Medical Literature. A Manual for Evidence-Based Clinical Practice. Chicago: AMA Press, 2002.

12 Levine MN, Gafni A, Markham B, MacFarlane D. A bedside decision instrument to elicit a patient's preference concerning adjuvant chemotherapy for breast cancer. Ann Intern Med 1992; 117: 53–8.

13   Nease RF, Kneeland T, O'Connor GT, et al. Variation in patient utilities for outcomes of the management of chronic stable angina: implications for clinical practice guidelines. JAMA 1995; 273: 1185–90.

14   Davis D, Evans M, Jadad A, et al. The case for knowledge translation: shortening the journey from evidence to effect. BMJ 2003; 327: 33–5.

We cannot pick up a newspaper or "surf the net" without being bombarded with concerns about potentially harmful interventions. These concerns lead to the posing of questions by both us and our patients, such as: Does living close to hydroelectric power lines increase the risk of cancer?, Do statins cause cancer?, Does exposure to aluminum cause Alzheimer's dementia?, Do elevated homocysteine levels cause coronary artery disease? And, we must make judgments about whether these medical interventions and environmental agents could be harmful to our patients.

To make these judgments, we need to be able to evaluate evidence about causation for its validity, importance, and direct relevance to our patients. Assessing the validity of the evidence is crucial if we are to avoid drawing the false-positive conclusion that an agent does cause an adverse event when, in truth, it does not, or the false-negative conclusion that an agent does not cause an adverse event when, in truth, it does. Clinical disagreements about whether a given patient has had an adverse drug reaction are not uncommon, and just because an adverse event occurred during treatment, it does not inevitably follow that the adverse event occurred because of that treatment.

The guides in Table 6.1 can help us to appraise the validity of an article about a putative harmful agent. We'll consider the following clinical scenario to illustrate our discussion.

6

> **Table 6.1** Is this evidence about harm valid?
>
> 1. Were there clearly defined groups of patients, similar in all important ways other than exposure to the treatment or other cause?
> 2. Were treatments/exposures and clinical outcomes measured in the same ways in both groups? (Was the assessment of outcomes either objective or blinded to exposure?)
> 3. Was the follow-up of the study patients sufficiently long (for the outcome to occur) and complete?
> 4. Do the results of the harm study fulfill some of the diagnostic tests for causation?
>   - Is it clear that the exposure preceded the onset of the outcome?
>   - Is there a dose–response gradient?
>   - Is there any positive evidence from a "dechallenge–rechallenge" study?
>   - Is the association consistent from study to study?
>   - Does the association make biological sense?

CLINICAL SCENARIO

During a routine health maintenance visit, we see a 45-year-old woman who complains of urge incontinence which has gotten progressively worse over the last 2 years, significantly impacting on her quality of life. Her past history is remarkable for three pregnancies (she had urge incontinence associated with each of these), and forceps were used during two of the births. She takes lorazepam occasionally at night for difficulty sleeping. She is on no other medications and has no smoking history. Her caffeine intake consists of 750 mL (25 oz) of coffee per day. Her clinical examination is unremarkable except for visible urine leakage when she is asked to cough while in the lithotomy position. Her post-void residual urine volume is 20 mL and a urinalysis is unremarkable. She recently read in the paper that caffeine can cause urinary incontinence and wants to know if this is true or if there are other factors that could be contributing to her problem.

In response to this scenario, we posed the question: In a woman with urge incontinence, does caffeine consumption cause urinary incontinence? Using the Clinical Queries function of PubMed we were able to identify an article that might help us to answer this question.[1]

TYPES OF REPORTS ON HARM/ETIOLOGY

As we discovered in Chapter 5, ideally the best evidence that we can find about the effects of therapy (and putative harmful agents) comes from systematic reviews. Individual randomized trials are seldom large enough to detect rare adverse events with precision—emphasizing the need to search for a systematic review. A systematic review that combines all relevant randomized trials or cohort studies might provide us with sufficiently large numbers of patients to detect even rare adverse events. When assessing the validity of such a systematic review, we need to consider the guides in Table 6.1 as well as those in Table 5.9. Unfortunately, such reviews aren't common, thus the discussion in this chapter will focus on randomized trials, cohort, case–control studies, and cross-sectional studies.

ARE THE RESULTS OF THIS HARM/ETIOLOGY STUDY VALID?

1. Were there clearly defined groups of patients, similar in all important ways other than exposure to the treatment or other cause?

Ideally, our search would yield a systematic review or a randomized trial in which women had been allocated, by a system analogous to tossing a coin, to caffeine (amount of caffeine could be specified) consumption (the top row in Table 6.2, whose total is $a + b$), or some comparison intervention (decaffeinated beverages) or placebo (the bottom row in Table 6.2, whose total is $c + d$) and then followed over time for the development of urinary incontinence. Randomization would tend to make the two treatment groups identical for all other causes of urinary incontinence (and we'd look for baseline differences in other putative causal agents between the groups), so we'd likely consider any statistically significant increase in urge

Table 6.2 Studies of whether caffeine consumption causes urinary incontinence

	Adverse outcome		
	Present (case)	Absent (controls)	Totals
Exposed to treatment (RCT or cohort)	a	b	a + b
Not exposed to treatment (RCT or cohort)	c	d	c + d
Totals	a + c	b + d	a + b + c + d

incontinence (adjusted for any important baseline differences) in the intervention group to be valid. Randomized control trials, however, are ill-suited (in size, duration, and ethics) for evaluating most uncommon possible harmful exposures, and we often have to make do with evidence from other types of studies. Consider how tough it would be to complete a study in which we randomize women to caffeine consumption vs. no caffeine consumption; and, returning to the questions posed at the beginning of this chapter, it would be impossible to randomize families to live in a house either close to or at a distance from power lines to determine the impact on cancer development! Unfortunately, the validity of the study designs used to detect harm is inversely proportional to their feasibility.

In the first of these alternatives, a cohort study, a group of participants who are exposed (a + b) to the treatment (or putative harmful agent) and a group or participants who aren't exposed (c + d) to it are followed for the development of the outcome of interest ("a" or "c"). Returning to our example, a cohort study would include a group of women with a history of caffeine consumption and a group without; then the risk of urge incontinence would be determined in each. As we discussed in Chapter 5, in observational studies such as cohort studies, the decision to prescribe and accept exposure is based on the patient's and/or physician's preferences and it is not randomized. As a result, "exposed" patients may differ from "non-exposed" patients in important determinants of the outcome (such determinants are called "confounders").* For example, consider a paper that looks at the relationship between estrogen use and the risk of urinary incontinence. Increasing age is associated with urinary incontinence and older women may be more likely to be using estrogen. Therefore age could be a confounder when comparing the risk of urinary incontinence in women using and not using estrogen. Investigators must document the characteristics of both cohorts of patients and either demonstrate their comparability or adjust for the confounders they identify (using special statistical techniques such as multivariable analysis). Of course, adjustments can only be made for confounders that are already known and have been measured, so we have to be careful when interpreting cohort studies.†

If the outcome of interest is rare or takes a long time to develop (e.g. the development of cancer or asbestosis), even large cohort studies may not be feasible and we will have to look for alternatives, such as case–control studies. In this study design, people with the outcome of interest (a + c) are identified as "cases" and those without it (b + d) are selected as "controls"; the proportion of each group who were exposed to the putative agent—i.e. $a/(a + c)$ or $b/(b + d)$—is assessed retrospectively. There is even more potential for confounding with case–control studies than with cohort studies because confounders that are transient or lead to early death won't even be able to be measured. For example, if patients are selected from hospital sources, the relationship between outcome and exposure will be distorted if patients who are exposed are more likely to be admitted to the hospital than are the unexposed. This was illustrated nicely in a systematic review that looked at the association between vasectomy and prostate cancer: the relative risk of prostate

---

* Confounders have the three properties of being: extraneous to the question posed; determinants of the outcome; and unequally distributed between exposed and non-exposed participants.

† As we mentioned in Chapter 5, this is another great thing about randomization: it balances the groups for confounders that we haven't identified yet!

cancer following vasectomy was elevated in hospital-based studies but not in population-based ones.

Inappropriate selection of control participants can lead to false associations, and "control" participants should have the same opportunity for exposure to the putative agent as the "case" participants. For example, if we found a case–control study evaluating the association between benzodiazepines and urinary incontinence that assembled women with urinary incontinence as cases but excluded patients with a history of falls or anxiety disorder from the control group (who might be at increased risk of exposure to benzodiazepines), we'd be right to wonder whether an observed association was spurious.

We can see that this study design easily lends itself to the exploration of possible relationships between many exposures and the outcome of interest (especially with the common usage and availability of administrative databases). Therefore we must bear in mind that, if a large number of potential associations are explored, a statistically significant finding could be based on chance alone.

When we're searching for an answer to an etiology question, the articles that we most commonly find describe cross-sectional studies; unfortunately, such studies are susceptible to even more bias than case–control studies. In a cross-sectional study, the authors would look at a group of women with urge incontinence $(a + c)$ and a group without $(b + d)$ and assess caffeine consumption ("a" or "b") in both. Exposure and outcomes are measured at the same time, and this highlights one of the major problems with this study type: which came first? Also, as with cohort and case–control studies, adjustment must be made for confounders.

Finally, we may only find case reports of one patient (or a case series of a few patients) who developed an adverse event while receiving the suspected treatment (cell "a" in Table 6.2). If the outcome is unusual and dramatic enough (phocomelia in children born to women who took thalidomide), such case reports and case series may be enough to answer our question. But, because these studies lack comparison groups, they are usually only sufficient for hypothesis generation and thus highlight the need for other studies.

We usually find information about the study type and how participants were selected in the abstract and methods sections of the article. Information describing participants is often found in the results section.

> The article that we found describes a case–control study that established a group of women with detrusor instability and a group without, and assessed caffeine consumption in both groups. Detrusor instability was diagnosed if the women had symptoms of urge incontinence and had evidence of bladder contraction and leakage on urodynamic testing. Control participants had stress incontinence; ideally, we'd want the control group to include age-matched continent women.

2. Were treatments/exposures and clinical outcomes measured in the same ways in both groups? (Was the assessment of outcomes either objective or blinded to exposure?)

We should place greater confidence in studies in which treatment exposures and clinical outcomes were measured in the same way in both groups. Moreover, we would prefer that the outcomes assessors were blind to the exposure in cohort studies and to the outcome and study hypothesis in case–control studies. Consider a report describing a cohort study looking at the association between coffee consumption and urinary incontinence. We'd be concerned if the investigator searched more aggressively for urinary incontinence in women who were known to have heavy caffeine consumption. Indeed, when the outcomes assessors aren't blinded to the exposure, they may search harder for the disease in the exposed group and identify disease that might otherwise have been unnoticed. Now consider a case–control study evaluating the same potential association; if the investigator is not blind to the outcome or study hypothesis, they might look harder for a history of heavy caffeine consumption in women whom they know to have urinary incontinence. Similarly, women with urinary incontinence might have considered their situation more carefully and may have greater ability or incentive to recall possible exposure. Thus, we'd feel more assured about the study if the report described that the patients (and their interviewers!) were blinded to the study hypothesis.

This discussion raises another, finer, point regarding the source of the information about the outcome or exposure of interest. Sometimes in articles we find that the investigators use medical records to seek information about the exposure or outcome retrospectively, and, as clinicians who complete these records (and often have to use them at a later date to dictate a discharge summary!), we have to ask ourselves if we consider this method sufficiently accurate. Consider, for example, the impact on a study's results if the likelihood of the data being recorded differs between the groups. Similarly, information from some administrative databases might not be as accurate as that collected prospectively (although, for certain types of information such as drug usage, a drug claims database will provide more accurate information than patient or physician recall!).

> Information about measurement of the exposure or outcome is usually included in the methods and results sections. In the study that we found, participants in both the control and the case groups were asked to complete a 48-hour voiding diary before urodynamic testing. This diary consisted of a structured intake and output diary to record the type and amount of fluid. They were asked to record their intake of coffee, tea, cola, and cocoa using a measuring cup. The reproducibility of this diary was assessed in a random sample of women after an interval of 1 week. It does not state if the patients were aware of the study hypothesis. Medical charts were reviewed to obtain information about potential confounders, including parity and smoking history.

3. Was the follow-up of the study patients sufficiently long (for the outcome to occur) and complete?

Ideally, we'd like to see that no patients were lost to follow-up because these patients may have had outcomes that would affect the conclusions of the study (in a cohort study looking at the association between urinary incontinence and caffeine consumption, imagine the impact on its results if a large number of women in the caffeine cohort left the study; we wouldn't know if it was because they developed urge incontinence and left the study to seek treatment, or because they became frustrated with the study). As mentioned in Chapter 5, evidence-based journals of secondary publication such as *ACP Journal Club* and *Evidence Based Medicine* use a 20% loss to follow-up as an exclusion criterion because it would be rare for a study to suffer such a loss and not to have its results affected. And, we'd like to see that the patients were followed for an appropriate period of time. For example, if we found a study of the association between Alzheimer's dementia and aluminum exposure that followed patients for only a few weeks, we wouldn't be able to distinguish a true- from a false-negative association.

4. Do the results of the harm study satisfy some of the diagnostic tests for causation?

Investigators may identify an association between an exposure and outcome, but is the exposure causative? There are a few "diagnostic tests for causation" that can help us with this concern, including the following:

Is it clear that the exposure preceded the onset of the outcome?
We'd want to make sure that the exposure (e.g. caffeine) occurred prior to the development of the adverse outcome (e.g. urinary incontinence).

Is there a dose–response gradient?
The demonstration of an increasing risk (or severity) of the adverse event with increasing exposure (increased dose and/or duration) to the putative causal agent strengthens the association. For example, in a recent case–control study looking at the association between homocysteine and ischemic heart disease, for each 5 μmmol/L increase in serum homocysteine level, there was a corresponding increase in the risk of ischemic heart disease.[2] In the

case–control study that we found looking at caffeine consumption and urinary incontinence, people with greater caffeine consumption (>400 mg/day) had a higher risk of urinary incontinence than those with lower caffeine consumption.

Is there any positive evidence from a "dechallenge–rechallenge" study?

We'd like to see that the adverse outcome decreases or disappears when the treatment is withdrawn and worsens or reappears when it is reintroduced. Returning to our clinical scenario, it would be useful to know that, if caffeine consumption is reduced or stopped, does the urinary incontinence improve in the heavy caffeine users? This information is not available from the study.

Is the association consistent from study to study?

If we were able to find multiple studies, or, better yet, a systematic review of the question, we could determine whether the association between exposure and the adverse event is consistent from study to study. For example, a recent systematic review looked at the association between serum homocysteine levels and ischemic heart disease and retrieved 30 relevant studies.[3] Interestingly, the authors noted that the retrospective studies that used population controls found a strong association, but that the prospective studies observed a less impressive association. Unfortunately, we weren't able to find additional recent studies looking at caffeine consumption and urinary incontinence.

Does the association make biological sense?

If the association between exposure and outcome makes biological sense (in terms of pathophysiology, etc.), a causal interpretation becomes more plausible. The authors of our study theorize that caffeine has an excitatory effect on detrusor smooth muscle, possibly through the release of intracellular calcium. (Keep in mind that this theory is based on data from animal models!)

ARE THE VALID RESULTS OF THIS HARM STUDY IMPORTANT?

If the study we find fails to satisfy the first three minimum standards in Table 6.1, we'd probably be better off abandoning it and continuing our search. But if we are satisfied that it meets these minimum guides, we need to decide if the association between exposure and outcome is sufficiently strong and convincing for us to do something about it. By this, we mean looking at the risk or odds of the adverse effect with (as opposed to without) exposure to the treatment; the higher the risk or odds, the stronger the association and the more we should be impressed by it. We can use the guides in Table 6.3 to determine if the valid results of the study are important.

Table 6.3 Are the valid results of this harm study important?

1. What is the magnitude of the association between the exposure and outcome?

2. What is the precision of the estimate of the association between the exposure and the outcome?

1. What is the magnitude of the association between the exposure and outcome?

As noted above, questions of etiology can be answered by several different study designs. Different study designs require different methods for estimating the strength of association between exposure to the putative cause and the outcome of interest. In randomized trials and cohort studies, this association is often described by calculating the risk (or incidence) of the adverse event in the exposed (or treated) patients relative to that in the unexposed (or untreated) patients. This relative risk (RR) is calculated as: $[a/(a + b)]/[c/(c + d)]$ (from Table 6.2). For example, if 1000 patients receive a treatment and 20 of them develop the outcome of interest:

$$a = 20$$
$$a/(a + b) = 2\%$$

If 1000 patients didn't receive the treatment and two experienced the outcome:

$$c = 2$$
$$c/(c + d) = 0.2\%$$

Therefore RR becomes:

$$2\%/0.2\% = 10$$

This means that patients receiving the treatment are 10 times more likely to experience the outcome as patients not receiving the treatment.

From the preceding example we can see that to calculate the RR we needed a group of treated participants and a group who didn't receive treatment; then we determined the proportion with the outcome in each. But, in case–control studies, we can't calculate the RR because the investigator selects the people with the outcomes (rather than those with the exposure) and we can't calculate the "incidence". Instead, we look to an indirect estimate of the strength of association in a case–control study; this is called an "odds ratio" (or relative odds) and (referring to Table 6.2) it is calculated as "ad/bc".

If, for example, 100 cases of patients with urge incontinence are identified and it's found that 90 of them had a history of caffeine consumption, then $a = 90$ and $c = 10$. If 100 patients without the outcome are assembled and it is found that 45 of them received the exposure, then $b = 45$ and $d = 55$ and the OR becomes:

$$OR = ad/bc$$
$$= (90 \times 55)/(45 \times 10)$$
$$= 11$$

This means that the odds of experiencing the adverse event for people who had a history of caffeine consumption was 11 times that of those who didn't have the same exposure.

OR and RR values >1 indicate that there is an increased risk of the adverse outcome associated with the exposure. And, when the RR = 1 or OR = 1, the adverse event is no more likely to occur with than without the exposure to the suspected agent. (Conversely, when the ORs and RRs <1, the adverse event is less likely to occur with the exposure to the putative agent than without.) It should also be noted that, when event rates are very low, the RR and OR approximate each other. And, they are close when the treatment effect is small. This is sometimes a cause for confusion because often in articles we find ORs have been calculated but that the authors report and discuss them as RRs.

How big should the RR or OR be for us to be impressed? This brings us back a bit into issues of validity, because we have to consider the strength of the study design when we're evaluating the strength of the association. As we discussed earlier in this chapter, a well-done randomized trial is susceptible to less bias than either a cohort or case–control study. Therefore, we'd be satisfied with a smaller increase in risk from a randomized trial than from a cohort or case–control study. Because cohort and, even more so, case–control studies are susceptible to many biases, we want to ensure that the OR is greater than that which would result from bias alone. We might not want to label an OR from a case–control study as impressive unless it is >4 for minor adverse events, and we'd set this value at progressively lower levels as the severity of the adverse event increases. There is less potential bias in cohort studies and therefore we might regard a relative risk of >3 as convincing for more severe adverse events.

Professor Les Irwig has provided another useful tip when looking at the strength of the association. It requires us to find a report that includes some adjustment for potential confounders. He suggests that we compare the unadjusted measure of association with one in which at least one known confounder has been adjusted out. If this adjustment produces a large decline in the RR or OR, we should be suspicious of a spurious association. If, in contrast, the adjusted OR or RR is stable with this adjustment, or if it rises rather than falls, our confidence in the validity of the association would be greater.

> In our study, high caffeine intake was associated with detrusor instability, but this OR declined slightly after adjusting for smoking history and age (OR 2.7 vs. 2.4 after adjustment).

Although the OR and RR tell us about the strength of the association, we need to translate this into some measure that is useful and intelligible both to us and to our patient. This is of particular importance when the discussion concerns a medication or some other medical intervention we and our patient are considering. For this, we can turn to the NNH (number needed to harm), which tells us the "number of patients who need to be exposed to the putative causal agent to produce one additional harmful event". The NNH can be calculated directly from trials and cohort studies in a fashion analogous to the NNT, but this time as the reciprocal of the difference in adverse event rates:

$$NNH = 1/[a/(a + b)] - [c/(c + d)]$$

For an OR derived from a case–control study, the calculation is more complex (remember, we can't determine "incidence" directly in a case–control study). Its scary formula reads:

if OR <1:

$$1 - [PEER(1 - OR)]/PEER(1 - PEER)(1 - OR)$$

if OR >1:

$$1 + [PEER(OR - 1)]/PEER(1 - PEER)(OR - 1)$$

where PEER is the patient expected event rate (the adverse event rate among individuals who are not exposed to the putative cause). We've made this easier for you by cranking out some typical PEERs and ORs and summarizing them in Tables 6.4 and 6.5. As you can see from the tables, for different PEERs, the same OR can lead to very different NNHs; it is therefore important that we

Table 6.4 Translating odds ratios (ORs) to NNHs when OR<1

Patient expected event rate (PEER)	For odds ratio LESS than 1						
	0.9	0.9	0.7	0.6	0.5	0.4	0.3
0.05	209[a]	104	69	52	41	34	29[b]
0.10	110	54	36	27	21	18	15
0.20	61	30	20	14	11	10	8
0.30	46	22	14	10	8	7	5
0.40	40	19	12	9	7	6	4
0.50	38	18	11	8	6	5	4
0.70	44	20	13	9	6	5	4
0.90	101[c]	46	27	18	12	9	4[d]

[a] The relative risk reduction (RRR) here is 10%.
[b] The RRR here is 49%.
[c] The RRR here is 1%.
[d] The RRR here is 9%.
Adapted from John Geddes (personal communication, 1999).

Table 6.5 Translating odds ratios (ORs) to NNHs when OR>1

Patient expected event rate (PEER)	For odds ratio GREATER than 1						
	1.1	1.25	1.5	1.75	2	2.25	2.5
0.05	212	86	44	30	23	18	16
0.10	113	46	24	16	13	10	9
0.20	64	27	14	10	8	7	6
0.30	50	21	11	8	7	6	5
0.40	44	19	10	8	6	5	5
0.50	42	18	10	8	6	6	5
0.70	51	23	13	10	9	8	7
0.90	121	55	33	25	22	19	18

The numbers in the body of the table are the NNHs for the corresponding ORs at that particular PEER.
Adapted from John Geddes (personal communication, 1999).

do our best to estimate the PEER when calculating the NNH. For example, if the OR = 0.90 and the PEER = 0.005, the NNH would be 2000; but if the PEER = 0.40 (and the OR = 0.90), the NNH would be 40. We'll consider individual patients in further detail in the next section.

Practicing EBM in real-time
The above formula is scary and we don't use it very often. If the answer we're looking for isn't in Table 6.4, we use the EBM calculator to quickly convert an OR to an NNH. Firing up the EBM calculator on the website (www.cebm.utoronto.ca) or from the accompanying CD, we can insert our OR of 0.90 and our PEER of 0.005 and, at the click of a button, the NNH is calculated (see Figure 6.1). We can also download this calculator to our PDA (personal digital assistant) for quick usage.

2. What is the precision of the estimate of the association between the exposure and outcome?

In addition to looking at the magnitude of the RR or OR, we need to look at its precision by examining the confidence interval (CI) around it. Credibility is highest when the entire confidence interval is narrow and remains within a clinically importantly increased risk. Earlier in this chapter we mentioned a systematic review that found a significant association between serum homocysteine level and risk of ischemic heart disease. From this study, the adjusted OR for ischemic heart disease or stroke associated with a 25% lower serum homocysteine level was 0.89, with 95% CI 0.83 to 0.96. The upper limit of this confidence interval is the smallest estimate of the strength of the association, and this approximates 1! Similarly, if a study finds no association, the limits of the confidence interval could tell us if a potentially important positive result (indicating an association) has been excluded. In our caffeine study, the OR was 2.4 (adjusted for age and smoking) with 95% CI 1.1 to 6.5. Note that the lower limit of the confidence interval is close to 1 and, as you will recall, when the OR approximates 1, the adverse event is no

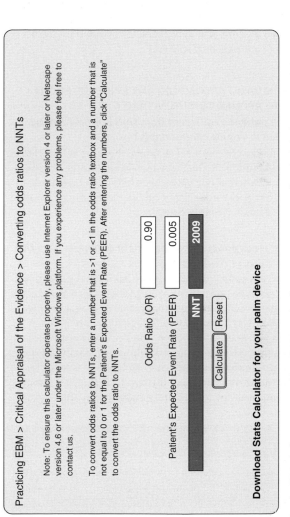

Practicing EBM > Critical Appraisal of the Evidence > Converting odds ratios to NNTs

Note: To ensure this calculator operates properly, please use Internet Explorer version 4 or later or Netscape version 4.6 or later under the Microsoft Windows platform. If you experience any problems, please feel free to contact us.

To convert odds ratios to NNTs, enter a number that is >1 or <1 in the odds ratio textbox and a number that is not equal to 0 or 1 for the Patient's Expected Event Rate (PEER). After entering the numbers, click "Calculate" to convert the odds ratio to NNTs.

Odds Ratio (OR) | 0.90

Patient's Expected Event Rate (PEER) | 0.005

NNT | 2009

[Calculate] [Reset]

Download Stats Calculator for your palm device

Figure 6.1 Using the EBM calculator to convert OR to NNH. Note that, because we are increasing the risk of a bad event, we calculate an NNH, not an NNT. This version of the calculator doesn't recognize the difference between NNT and NNH.

more likely to occur with than without the exposure to the suspected agent.

Once we have decided that the evidence we have found is both valid and important, we need to consider if it can be applied to our patient (Table 6.6).

CAN THIS VALID AND IMPORTANT EVIDENCE ABOUT HARM BE APPLIED TO OUR PATIENT?

1. Is our patient so different from those included in the study that its results cannot apply?

As emphasized in previous chapters, the issue is not whether our patient fulfills all the inclusion criteria for the study we found, but whether our patient is so different from those in the study that its results are of no help to us. See p. 136 for further discussion of this issue.

2. What is our patient's risk of benefit and harm from the agent?

To apply the results of a study to an individual patient, we need to estimate our patient's risk of the adverse event if she were not exposed to the putative cause. There's a hard way and an easy way to tackle this. The hard way requires searching for good evidence on prognosis; the much easier way requires estimating the risk relative to that of unexposed individuals in the study. Just as with NNTs in Chapter 5, we can express this as a decimal fraction (called "f"): if our patient is at half the risk of study patients, f = 0.5; if our

Table 6.6 Guides for deciding whether valid important evidence about harm can be applied to our patient

1. Is our patient so different from those included in the study that its results cannot apply?
2. What is our patient's risk of benefit and harm from the agent?
3. What are our patient's preferences, concerns, and expectations from this treatment?
4. What alternative treatments are available?

patient is at three times the risk, f = 3. The study NNH can then be divided by "f" to produce the NNH for our individual patient. For example, suppose a study found we'd only need to treat 150 people with a statin to cause one additional cancer. But if we think our patient is at twice the risk of the study patients, f = 2 and 150/2 generates an NNH of 75. If, on the other hand, we thought our patient was at one-third the risk (f = 0.33), the NNH for patients like ours becomes 455.

In situations such as this when we're considering the use of a medication, the NNH needs to be balanced against the corresponding NNT summarizing the benefit of this treatment. The resulting crude "likelihood of being helped vs. harmed" (LHH, see Ch. 5) by this treatment can provide the starting point for the last step, described in the next section.

3. What are our patient's preferences, concerns, and expectations from this treatment?

It is vital that we incorporate our patient's unique concerns and preferences into any shared decision-making process. In the case of potentially harmful therapy, and just as in Chapter 5, we can ask our patient to quantify her values for both the potential adverse event and the target event we hope to prevent with the proposed therapy. The result is a severity-adjusted likelihood of being helped or harmed by the therapy. If we are unsure of our patient's baseline risk, or if she is unsure about her values for the outcomes, a sensitivity analysis can be done. That is, different values for relative severity could be inserted, and we and our patient could determine at which point the decision would change.

4. What alternative treatments are available?

Finally, we and our patient could explore alternative management options. Is there another medication we could consider? Is there any effective non-pharmacological therapy available?

Returning to our patient and having reviewed the evidence about caffeine consumption and urge incontinence, she is considered to have heavy caffeine consumption. The bottom line from the study suggests that heavy caffeine consumption may increase the risk of detrusor instability, but this association appears weak. However, after discussion with our patient, she would like to consider this option further in an attempt to reduce her symptoms, and together we have outlined a proposal to look at an n-of-1 study to determine if a reduction in caffeine consumption will alleviate her symptoms (see Ch. 5 for detailed discussion of n-of-1 studies). We have also discussed other risk factors that were identified in studies and which may be contributing to her incontinence, including multiparity and history of forceps delivery. If no symptom resolution occurs with modification of caffeine consumption, we've agreed to consider a trial of pelvic floor muscle training which is a non-pharmacological intervention that has been proven to be beneficial in a recent systematic review.

PRACTICING EBM IN REAL-TIME

Formulating a question, and then retrieving, appraising, and applying relevant evidence from the primary literature will usually take longer than the average clinical appointment. There are several ways to tackle the time constraints, focusing on finding shortcuts to facilitate practicing EBM. As we've already mentioned (in Ch. 2), if we can find our answer in a high-quality pre-appraised resource, we're ahead of the game; but, unfortunately, many of these resources don't yet have a broad coverage of topics, so we may not find anything relevant. If we're lucky to have a local librarian or consultant pharmacist who can help us track down the evidence, we'd ask them for some help. Alternatively, we can share tasks with other colleagues, either locally or virtually using e-mail discussion groups. We'd also consider asking our patient to book a return visit in a week to review the evidence with them at that time, giving us some time to review the evidence between visits. If the same clinical issues arise commonly, we could develop our own patient information leaflets briefly summarizing some of the evidence. In the same way, we could keep our CATs (critically appraised topics) (with expiry dates!) on file for our own needs if we expect the clinical problem to arise again. Finally, depending on how interested our patient is in being part of the shared decision-making process, they could be involved in each step along the way.

A FINAL NOTE

Material in this chapter can be applied to questions about whether treatments do more harm than good, as well as to questions of causation around lifestyle issues such as caffeine consumption, and around environmental issues such as living close to hydroelectric power lines. The principles are all the same, but, in lifestyle issues, the harm is contrasted with the satisfaction or other gains derived from pursuing the putatively "unhealthy" practice. And with environmental issues, discussion must consider interventions to reduce the risk and their associated cost-effectiveness and feasibility.

REFERENCES

1 Arya LA, Myers DL, Jackson ND. Dietary caffeine intake and the risk for detrusor instability: a case–control study. Obstet Gynecol 2000; 96: 85–9.

2 Wald N, Watt HC, Law MR, et al. Homocysteine and ischemic heart disease: results of a prospective study with implications regarding prevention. Arch Intern Med 1998; 158: 862–7.

3 The Homocysteine Studies Collaboration. Homocysteine and the risk of ischemic heart disease and stroke: a meta analysis. JAMA 2002; 288: 2015–22.

Further reading

Guyatt G, Rennie D, eds. Users' Guides to the Medical Literature. Chicago: AMA Press, Chicago, 2002.

Sackett DL, Haynes RB, Guyatt GH, Tugwell P. Clinical Epidemiology. A Basic Science for Clinical Medicine, 2nd edn. Boston: Little, Brown, 1991.

Teaching methods

Throughout the book we've provided ideas for teaching methods when they fit with the themes of previous chapters (e.g. the "educational prescription" in Ch. 1); you can find them in the index, or by scanning the page margins for the mortar board icon. In this chapter, we've collected other ideas for teaching learners how to practice EBM. We'll describe three main modes for teaching EBM, consider some successes and failures with various teaching methods, and then examine some specific clinical teaching situations.

We're clinical teachers and collectors of teaching methods, not educational theorists. From what we've learned so far about theories of learning, rather than adhering strictly to one theory (e.g. behaviorism or constructivism), we find ourselves using ideas and methods from several schools of thought. To the delight of both our critics (who claim we're adrift in a *sans*-theoretical fog) and our colleagues (who know us better than that, and who wouldn't want to be bored), we'll skip building our own theory and concentrate instead on how we put the principles we've learned from others into practice. In developing as teachers, we've been most strongly influenced by the people who taught us, yet we've also been influenced by several works on teaching and learning.[1–11]

7

We'd like to draw upon high-quality evidence from educational research to guide our recommendations about what works and what doesn't in teaching EBM. However, as discussed in detail in Chapter 8, little research has been conducted to date on how best we can teach the knowledge, attitudes, and skills of practicing and teaching EBM. Thus, the suggestions in this chapter are primarily based on the teaching experiences we've had ourselves or collected from others.

THREE MODES OF TEACHING EBM

From what we've done, seen or heard about, we've noticed that although there may be as many ways to teach EBM as there are teachers, most of these methods fall into one of three categories or teaching modes: role-modeling evidence-based care; teaching clinical medicine using evidence; and teaching specific EBM skills (see Table 7.1).

Mode 1 involves role-modeling the practice of EBM. For example, when you and a learner see a hospitalized patient with upper extremity deep vein thrombosis, you might ask yourself aloud a question about the frequency of underlying causes of this disorder, admit aloud you don't know the answer, find and appraise evidence about this topic, and discuss aloud how you'll use the evidence in planning your diagnostic strategy. When we role-model evidence-based practice, our learners see us incorporating evidence with other knowledge into real-time clinical decisions, whether for individual patients or for groups of patients. Thus, learners

Table 7.1 Three modes of teaching EBM

1. Role-modeling evidence-based practice:

   a. Learners see evidence as part of good patient care.

   b. Teaching by example: "actions speak louder than words".

   c. Learners see us use judgment in integrating evidence into decisions.

2. Teaching clinical medicine with evidence:

   a. Learners see evidence as part of good clinical learning.

   b. Teaching by weaving: evidence is taught along with other knowledge.

   c. Learners see us use judgment in integrating evidence with other knowledge.

3. Teaching specific EBM skills:

   a. Learners learn how to understand evidence and use it wisely.

   b. Teaching by coaching: learners get explicitly coached as they develop.

   c. Learners see us use judgment as we carry out the five steps with them (asking, searching, appraising, applying, and evaluating).

come to see the use of evidence as part of good patient care, not something separate from it. We show by our example that we really do it, when we really do it, and how we really do it.

Mode 2 involves adding the results of clinical care research to other things you teach about a clinical topic. For instance, when you and a learner examine a patient with congestive heart failure, after teaching how to hear the S3 gallop using the stethoscope's bell, you can summarize research results about this finding's accuracy and precision as a test for heart failure. When we include research evidence in what we teach about clinical medicine, our learners see us integrating evidence from clinical care research with knowledge from other sources: the biology of human health and disease, the medical humanities, the understanding of systems of health care, the values and preferences of patients, and our clinical expertise. Learners come to see the use of evidence as part of good clinical learning, not something separate from it. By weaving evidence into the mix of knowledge we teach from, we can show specifically when and how evidence can inform various clinical decisions.

Mode 3 involves explicitly teaching specific skills of EBM. For instance, when learning about the care of a patient facing newly diagnosed ovarian cancer, in addition to teaching the "content" of this cancer's prognosis, you can also teach your team members the "process" of how to find and critically appraise studies of prognosis. When we teach specific EBM skills, we show our learners how the wise use of evidence fits into the broader context of lifelong clinical learning. As clinical teachers, we aim to help our learners develop a critical and reflective stance when considering, not only evidence from clinical care research, but also when examining knowledge from any source. The Cochrane Review on teaching critical appraisal skills[12] found some trial evidence that teaching critical appraisal improves participants' knowledge, but no evidence about impact on patient outcomes or about which methods are most effective.

We use all three modes of teaching EBM in our work, moving from one to another to fit the clinical and teaching circumstances. Since each mode requires somewhat different preparation and may draw upon differing strengths and weaknesses, we may begin our teaching careers feeling more comfortable with one mode than with the others. Yet since good teachers of EBM (or anything else for that matter) are made, not born, it is through deliberate practice of, and purposeful reflection on, each mode that we can refine our teaching skills. Although no mode is inherently more "right" than any other, we find that using evidence in our practice and teaching (Modes 1 and 2) gives us more legitimacy and realism when we teach our learners about the specific EBM skills (Mode 3).

TEACHING EBM: TOP 10 SUCCESSES

Reflecting on what worked well can help refine one's teaching;[13] here we describe methods in which teaching EBM (Table 7.2) has been successful for us or for others.

Table 7.2 The top 10 successes we've had or seen in teaching EBM

Teaching EBM succeeds:

1. When it centers around real clinical decisions and actions.

2. When it focuses on learners' actual learning needs.

3. When it balances passive ("diastolic") with active ("systolic") learning.

4. When it connects "new" knowledge to "old" (what learners already know).

5. When it involves everyone on the team.

6. When it attends to both the feelings and the knowing of learning.

7. When it matches, and takes advantage of, the clinical setting, available time, and other circumstances.

8. When it balances preparedness with opportunism.

9. When it makes explicit how to make judgments, whether about the evidence itself or about how to integrate evidence with other knowledge, clinical expertise, and patient preferences.

10. When it builds learners' lifelong learning abilities.

---

1. When it centers around real clinical decisions and actions

Since practicing EBM begins and ends with patients, it shouldn't surprise you that our most enduring and successful efforts in teaching EBM have been those that centered on the illnesses of patients directly under the care of our learners. The clinical needs of these patients serve as the starting point for identifying our knowledge needs and asking answerable clinical questions that are directly relevant to these needs. By returning to our patients' problems after searching and appraising evidence about them, we can demonstrate how to integrate evidence with other knowledge and our patients' preferences and unique circumstances. If the learning group members are not on the same clinical service and don't share responsibility for the same patients, we can still engage the group in discussing one or more real clinical decisions they've previously faced or expect to face in the future. Using this method, learners see the use of evidence in its natural context.

2. When it focuses on learners' actual learning needs

We think teaching means helping learners learn, and we think of ourselves as guides or coaches of learning. Since clinical learners will vary widely in their motivations, their starting knowledge, their learning styles and skills, their learning contexts and available time for learning, we may need to employ a wide variety of teaching strategies and tactics. One size does not fit all, so in our teaching practices we need the skills to accurately assess our learners' developmental stage, diagnose their learning needs, and select appropriate teaching interventions. We need to adjust our teaching to match our learners' developmental stage and the pace of their understanding. Since many of our learners will also have other demands they must satisfy, such as passing written exams, we need to acknowledge these conflicting demands, help learners cope with them, and adjust our teaching to fit the circumstances.

3. When it balances passive ("diastolic") with active ("systolic") learning

Learning clinical medicine has been described using an analogy to the cardiac cycle, with passive learning devices such as listening to a lecture compared with diastolic filling and active learning devices compared with systolic pumping.[14] Both kinds of learning are useful, and both work best when used in balance with each other. Since most learners arrive on our clinical teams having had much more experience with passive learning than active (for some, this excess is measured in decades!), we find ourselves strongly emphasizing active learning strategies. Besides, while passive techniques may be effective for learning some kinds of knowledge (the "know what"), only through active learning can we learn how to put this knowledge into action (the "know how").

4. When it connects "new" knowledge to "old" (what learners already know)

By the time they arrive on our clinical teams, learners usually have very large funds of knowledge, of both experiential and book learning. Whether teaching in Modes 1, 2, or 3, with questions we can stimulate learners to recall knowledge from memory, which activates this knowledge for use and also helps us identify any knowledge gaps or misunderstandings. By connecting the new information we teach to their existing fact networks, we help learners comprehend the new lessons better and put them in context. We also help learners reorganize their knowledge into schemes more useful for clinical decision-making.

5. When it involves everyone on the team

When we as teachers divide the work of learning into chunks so that everyone can be involved, we help the team in four ways. First, a broader range of questions can be asked and answered, since the work can be shared by several people. Second, when seniors pair up with juniors to help them track down and appraise answers, their capacity for teamwork is reinforced. Third, since every team member can benefit from each team member's efforts, sharing lessons across the team multiplies the learning yields. Fourth, the team's interactive discussions as they learn can help individual team members clarify misconceptions, consolidate the lessons learned, and consider their implications for decision and action. Involving everyone needn't mean that all are assigned equal amounts of work: educational prescriptions can be handed out in differing amounts, depending on learners' other work loads.

6. When it attends to both the feelings and the knowings of learning

As we mentioned in Chapter 1, learning can involve strong emotions, whether "positive", such as the joy of discovery or the fun of learning with others, or "negative", such as the fear of being asked a question, the shame of not knowing an answer, or the anger when learning time is squandered. We can help learners grow in learning effectiveness by helping them acknowledge the feelings of learning and developing appropriate, rather than maladaptive, responses. We can also help learners by showing some of our own feelings, such as our enthusiasm for learning. Next, recall that making sound clinical decisions requires us to draw upon different kinds of knowledge, developed through different ways of knowing: we develop clinical expertise through experience with patient care and with coaching; we develop knowledge of our patients' perspectives and preferences through conversation and working with them; and we develop knowledge of research results through reading and critical appraisal. We can help our learners grow in learning effectiveness by identifying these different sources of knowing as we teach, and by coaching them to refine their abilities to know and learn in each way.

7. When it matches, and takes advantage of, the clinical setting, available time, and other circumstances

Each patient situation and clinical setting define a different learning context, where things such as the severity of illness, the pace of the work, the available time, and person-power all combine to determine what can be learned and when, where, how, and by whom it is learned. Teaching tactics that work well in one setting (e.g. the outpatient clinic) may not fit at all in other settings (e.g. the intensive care unit). We can improve patient- and learner-centered learning by capitalizing on the opportunities that present themselves in these different settings and circumstances *as they occur.*

8. *When it balances preparedness with opportunism*

We can anticipate many of the questions our learners will ask, since they'll arise from the patients, health states, and clinical decisions we encounter frequently in our teaching settings. To prepare for these opportunities, we can gather, appraise, and summarize the evidence we'll use to inform those decisions, then place these summaries at or near the sites of care. By being well prepared, we need only recognize the clinical situations when (not if) they occur, seize the teaching moment, and guide the learners in understanding and using the evidence. This kind of opportunism can be supplemented by another kind: recognizing teaching opportunities among questions for which we haven't prepared ahead, to model and involve learners in the steps of asking questions, finding and appraising evidence, and integrating it into our clinical decisions.

9. *When it makes explicit how to make judgments, whether about the evidence itself or about how to integrate evidence with other knowledge, clinical expertise, and patient preferences and circumstances*

As the previous chapters show, practicing EBM requires us to use judgment when choosing questions, when selecting knowledge resources, when appraising evidence critically, and when integrating the evidence into clinical decisions. Using judgment requires not only that we be able to sort, weigh, and integrate knowledge of different kinds, but also that we reflect on the underlying values made visible by our choices. Learning to make these judgments wisely takes time and practice, so it seems sensible to make this practice deliberate and these discussions explicit.

10. When it builds learners' lifelong learning abilities

Clinical practice can be thought of as the ultimate open-book test, occurring daily over a lifetime of practice, with the entire world's knowledge potentially available as "the book" for clinicians to use. To develop and sustain the skills to use this knowledge wisely, learners need hard work and coaching, concentrating on such things as reflectiveness (to recognize their own learning needs) resilience (to respond adaptively to their cognitive dissonance), and resourcefulness (to know how to carry out learning on their own). One of the best ways we know of to stimulate this process is to make learning multistaged. When we divide the learning into manageable chunks and plan its achievement over several stages, we allow learners to try their hands at each stage, coming to the next encounter with both the learning yield and with experiences that can guide new learning objectives. Multistaged learning also helps with managing time well, because on busy clinical services it is usually easier to schedule several short appointments for learning rather than one large block.

TEACHING EBM: TOP 10 FAILURES

To compare with these successes, we collect here ten mistakes we've either made or seen in teaching EBM (Table 7.3), since reflecting on failures can also help refine one's teaching.[15]

The first two mistakes happen when experts in any field of basic science hold the notion that in order to pragmatically apply the fruits of a science learners have to master its methods of inquiry. This is demonstrably untrue (doctors save the lives of patients with heart failure by prescribing them beta-blockers, not by learning how to measure the number of beta-receptors in cardiac muscle cells). It is also counterproductive, for it requires learners who want to become clinicians to learn the skills of transparently foreign careers, and we shouldn't be surprised by learners' indifference and hostility to courses in statistics, epidemiology, and the like. Our recognition of these mistakes explains why there is so little about statistics in

Table 7.3 The top 10 mistakes we've made or seen in teaching EBM

Teaching EBM fails:

1. When learning how to do research is emphasized over how to use it.

2. When learning how to do statistics is emphasized over how to interpret them.

3. When teaching EBM is limited only to finding flaws in published research.

4. When teaching portrays EBM as substituting research evidence for, rather than adding it to, clinical expertise, patient values, and circumstances.

5. When teaching with or about evidence is disconnected from the team's learning needs about either their patients' illnesses or their own clinical skills.

6. When the amount of teaching exceeds the available time or the learners' attention.

7. When teaching occurs at the speed of the teacher's speech or mouse clicks, rather than at the pace of the learners' understanding.

8. When the teacher strives for full educational closure by the end of each session, rather than leaving plenty to think about and learn between sessions.

9. When it humiliates learners for not already knowing the "right" fact or answer.

10. When it bullies learners to decide or act based on fear of others' authority or power, rather than on authoritative evidence and rational argument.

this book (and most of that in an appendix), and why our emphasis is on how to use research reports, not how to generate them.

The third and fourth mistakes can occur when any narrow portion of a complex undertaking is inappropriately emphasized to the exclusion of all other portions. In response, learners may develop skills in one step of EBM, such as the ability to find study flaws in critical appraisal, but don't develop any other skills. This hurts learners in two ways. First, by seeing modeled an unbalanced approach to appraising evidence, learners can develop protracted nihilism (see Table 7.11), a powerful *de*-motivator of evidence-based learning. Second, without learning to follow critical appraisal by integrating evidence sensibly into clinical decisions, learners aren't prepared to act independently on evidence in the future (when their teachers are gone), so they are dependent on others to interpret evidence for them and to tell them how to act.

The fifth mistake can happen in several ways, such as when we fail to begin and end our teaching sessions with the learners' patients, when we fail to diagnose either the patients' clinical needs or our learners' resulting learning needs, or when we fail to connect our teaching to our learners' motivations, career plans, or stage of development as clinicians. The resulting disconnect between what we teach and what the learners need to learn usually means, not only that the learners won't retain anything we do cover, but also that we consume the available learning time before they can learn what they really needed. As such foregone learning opportunities accumulate, our learners fall behind their peers in developing clinical excellence and lifelong learning skills.

The sixth and seventh mistakes occur when the teacher over-estimates the amount that should be covered in the available time. Although teachers' motives needn't be evil—these mistakes can arise simply out of enthusiasm for the subject—the resulting overly long and/or overly fast presentation taxes the learners' abilities to register, comprehend, or retain the material covered.

The eighth mistake happens when we behave as if learning only occurs during formal teaching sessions. This behavior is harmful in two ways. First, it cuts off problem-solving during the sessions themselves ("We're running out of time, so I want to stop this discussion and give you the right answers"). Second, it prevents or impairs the development of the self-directed learning skills that will be essential for our learners' continuing professional development.

The ninth and tenth entries are included here because they are still commonplace among medical education programs, and at some of these institutions they remain a source of twisted pride. Such treatment of learners by their teachers is not simply wrong in human terms, it is demonstrably counterproductive. First, the resulting shame and humiliation learners feel will strongly discourage the very learning that the teacher's ridicule was meant to stimulate. Second, in adapting to the rapid loss of trust and safety in the learning climate, learners will start employing strategies to hide their true learning needs and protect themselves from their teachers, undermining future learning and teaching efforts. Understandably, learners with prior experiences of these behaviors may be very reluctant to even start the practice of EBM by asking a question, since it exposes them to the potential threat of repeated abuse.*

Having considered these successes and failures, we'll turn next to ways to incorporate teaching EBM into some learning encounters that are commonly present in the education of clinicians in many countries. We'll then take two examples of these opportunities to explore them in more detail.

TEACHING AND LEARNING EBM ON AN INPATIENT SERVICE

There are at least seven different sorts of rounds that the authors have conducted (or survived) on an inpatient service; we've summarized them in Table 7.4. These rounds share several features, including severe constraints on learners' time and the innumerable interruptions. Little surprise, then, that for most of these types of rounds, much of our EBM teaching is through modeling evidence-based practice and teaching clinical topics with evidence Modes 1 and 2.

During rounds on newly admitted patients ("post-take" or "admission" rounds), there is usually time only for quick demonstrations of evidence-based bits of the clinical exam and how to get from pre-test to post-test probabilities of the

---

* Contrast this with the actions of colleague David Pencheon, who asks new medical students questions of increasing difficulty until they respond with "I don't know". Upon hearing these words, he rewards them with a box of Smarties and tells them that these are the three most important words in medicine.[16]

Table 7.4 Incorporating EBM into inpatient rounds

Type of round	Objectives[a]	Evidence of highest relevance	Restrictions[b]	Strategies
"Post-take" or admission rounds (after every period on call, all over the hospital, by post-call team and consultant)	Decide on working diagnosis and initial therapy of newly admitted patients	Accuracy and precision of the clinical examination and other diagnostic tests; efficacy and safety of initial therapy	Time, motion (can't stay in one spot), and fatigue of team post-call	Demonstrate evidence-based exam and getting from pre-test to post-test probability; carry a PDA or a loose-leaf book with synopses of evidence; write educational prescriptions; add a clinical librarian to the team
Morning report (every day, sitting down, by entire medical service)	Briefly review new patients and discuss and debate the process of evaluating and managing one or more of them	Accuracy and precision of the clinical examination and other diagnostic tests; efficacy and safety of initial therapy	Time	Educational prescriptions for foreground questions (and fact follow-ups for background questions); give 1–2-minute summaries of CATs
Work rounds (every day, on one or several wards, by trainees)	Examine every patient and determine their current clinical state; review and (re)order tests and treatments	Accuracy and precision of diagnostic tests; efficacy and safety of ongoing treatment, and interactions	Time and motion	In electronic records, create links between test results or treatment orders and the relevant evidence
Consultant walking rounds (1–3 times a week, on one or several wards, by trainees and consultant)	As in work rounds, but objectives vary widely by consultant	As in work rounds, plus those resulting from individual consultant's objectives	Time, relevance to junior members ("shifting dullness")	Model how to explain evidence to patients and incorporate into decisions (e.g. LHH)

Table 7.4 *(Cont'd)*

Type of round	Objectives[a]	Evidence of highest relevance	Restrictions[b]	Strategies
Review rounds (or "card-flip") (every day, sitting down and at the bedside, by trainees and consultants)	45-second reviews of each patient's diagnosis, treatment, progress, and discharge plans; identification of complicated patients who require bedside exam and more discussion	Wherever the educational prescriptions have led the learners	Time	Educational prescriptions for foreground questions (and fact follow-ups for background questions); give 1–2-minute summaries of critical appraisal; audit whether you are following through on evidence-based care
Social issues rounds (periodically, by trainees and a host of other professionals)	Review of each patient's status, discharge plan, referral, and post-hospital follow-up	Efficacy and safety of community services and social interventions	Time, availability of relevant participants, and enormous burden of paperwork	Ask other health professionals to provide synopses of evidence for what they routinely propose

Preceptor rounds ("pure education") (1–2 times a week, by learners (often stratified) and teacher)	Develop and improve skills for clinical examination and presentation	Accuracy and precision of the clinical examination	Time, teacher's energy, and other commitments	Practice presentations and feedback; use evidence about clinical exam; educational prescriptions for foreground questions (and fact follow-ups for background questions); give concise summaries on critical appraisal
"Down-time" or "dead space" during any round	Wait for the elevator or for a report or for a team member to show up, catch up, answer a page, get off the phone, find a chart, etc.	No limit	Imagination and ingenuity	Insert synopses of evidence, either from recent educational prescriptions (and fact follow-ups), or from pre-appraised evidence resources

aIncreasingly, all rounds include the objective of discharging patients as soon as possible.
bAll rounds require confidentiality when discussions of individual patients occur in public areas.

leading diagnosis (in about 2–5 minutes), or for introducing concise (one page, or 2–4 PDA screens) and instantly available (within <15 seconds) synopses of evidence about the key diagnostic and treatment decisions that have been, are being, or ought to be, carried out.

Can synopses of evidence really get there that fast? Yes, by using either or both of two strategies. First, anticipate the clinical decisions you're likely to encounter, then find (or make) concise synopses of the evidence that can inform those decisions and carry them with you. We've seen several formats used, including structured synopses on paper in a binder (Dave Sackett carried his "big red book", and one of us carries a "medicine consult notebook"),[17] on notebook computer carried by cart,[18] in portable textbook format (e.g. *Clinical Evidence* or *Evidence Based Acute Medicine*), or even more concise summaries carried in a PDA.[19] Second, as information technology advances, more of us may find ourselves working in health systems that provide instant electronic access, not only to unfiltered evidence resources such as PubMed, but also to filtered evidence resources, such as Cochrane Reviews, ACP Journal Club Online, Evidence-Based On Call, and Clinical Evidence, for both PCs and PDAs. Of course, when the evidence isn't so quickly to hand, we can write educational prescriptions to be filled after admission rounds, as we described in Chapter 1.

In many centers, the individual teams' post-take rounds are supplemented by a service-wide, sit-down "morning report". We'll return to introducing EBM in morning report later in this chapter.

"Work rounds", during which the team's trainees carry out the rapid, detailed, bedside review of patients' problems, and progress and the review and (re)ordering of their diagnostic tests and treatments, provide a challenging yet fruitful setting for teaching in modes 1 or 2. Most challenging perhaps is that the consultant/attending teacher is not present, yet the teacher can still influence the team's learning during these rounds, using the following three strategies. First, once the team has adopted the approach of integrating evidence into decisions when the attending is present, we can encourage its continued use by debriefing them on their successes and failures in applying evidence to decisions, and on questions they'd posed during work rounds, and by helping them to find evidence-based answers the whole team can use. Second, we can help our entire team get access to the evidence synopses we use when we are there, either by sharing them (e.g. "beaming" from our PDA to theirs), or by showing them how to access the resources themselves (e.g. providing URLs for filtered resources). Third, in some centers, the information systems that record patients' clinical data are linked to guidelines or summaries of evidence that can help team members take appropriate action. Note that these systems do not require learners to recognize their evidence needs, but supply it in the context of patients in their care, reinforcing the importance of the evidence and also recognizing that it's left to the clinician and the patient to decide on its implementation.

"Consultant walking rounds" provide an excellent opportunity for the consultant to model how to combine evidence with patients' values and expectations in making management decisions. For example, the consultant might take 5–10 minutes to demonstrate how to use the likelihood of being helped vs. harmed (LHH) by a treatment under consideration (the LHH was discussed in Ch. 5). These rounds also provide great opportunities to teach in mode 2, for example by incorporating evidence about the accuracy of findings of volume depletion along with teaching how to choose the initial intravenous fluid for a patient with hypovolemia.

Many consultants (some of whom keep note cards on each patient) lead short (<1 hour), frequent (e.g. daily, when not "on take") review rounds (sometimes called the "card flip") of all patients on the service. This has been most fruitful for us when we held it in a work/seminar room right on or near the wards. Patients are summarized in four quick phrases (what they've got, what we're doing about it, how they are doing, when and where they are going), and this quick review is interrupted for only two reasons. The first reason is when a patient is so sick or unstable or so problematic that he or she needs to be examined by the whole team. The second interruption is for evidence-based learning. These may be precipitated by any team member and are of three sorts: first, challenges (the more vigorous the better) to provide evidence that the evaluation or management decisions being made for a patient are valid and appropriate; second, quick responses, usually with evidence synopses, to earlier challenges from previous rounds; and third, very brief demonstrations of the critical appraisal or application of evidence to specific patients.

"Pure" education rounds are conducted after the patients have been cared for, and therefore enjoy the luxuries of relaxed time and choice of topic. Topics of special relevance to EBM include: the more thorough bedside evaluations of the techniques, accuracy, and precision of the clinical examination; more detailed learner-led discussions of how they found and appraised evidence; and the more detailed explanation and practice of skills such as generating patient-specific NNTs (number needed to treat) and NNHs (number needed to harm). When these rounds are directed to new clinical clerks, they can include mastery of the orderly and thorough presentation of patients on the service, along the lines shown in Table 7.5.

Finally, all rounds of teams of size "n" are peppered with "down-times" or "dead spaces" that interrupt the learning process and annoy at least n–1 of its members. Rather than permit learning to decelerate or be replaced by thoughts of lunch and sore backs, teachers can seize the moment and insert narrow "slices" of evidence (instead of the "whole pie") from a recent evidence-based journal or website visit, or perhaps from a previously prepared evidence synopsis. Because no learner wants to be excluded from receiving these learning slices, this tactic encourages team members to avoid causing future down-time.

TEACHING AND LEARNING EBM IN THE OUTPATIENT CLINIC

Time both hampers and favors teaching in the outpatient setting. On the one hand, individual outpatient

Table 7.5 A guide for learners presenting an "old" patient at follow-up rounds

The presentation should summarize 20 things in 2 minutes:

1. The patient's name.

2. The patient's age.

3. The patient's sex.

4. The patient's occupation/social role.

5. When the patient was admitted (or transferred) to the service.

6. The clinical problem(s) that led to admission (or transfer). (A clinical problem can be a symptom, a sign, a cluster of symptoms and signs, a clinical syndrome, an event, an injury, a test result, a diagnosis, a psychologic state, a social predicament, etc.)

7. The number of active problems the patient has at present

For each active problem:

8. Its most important symptoms, if any.

9. Its most important signs, if any.

10. The results of diagnostic tests or other evaluations.

11. The explanation (diagnosis or health state) for the problem.

12. The treatment plan instituted for the problem.

13. The response to this treatment plan.

14. The future and contingency plans for this problem.

[Repeat 8–14 for each active problem.]

15. Your plans for discharge, post-hospital care, and follow-up.

16. Whether you've filled the fact follow-up or educational prescription that you requested when this patient was admitted (in order to better understand the background of this patient's condition or the foreground of how best to care for this patient, respectively).

If so:

17. How you found the relevant evidence.

18. What you found: the clinical bottom line from that evidence.

19. Your critical appraisal of that evidence for its validity, importance, and applicability.

20. How that critically appraised evidence will alter your care of that (or the next similar) patient.

If not:

17a. When you are going to fill it.

appointments are short, constraining both the number and breadth of clinical and learning issues that can be addressed during any single visit. On the other hand, outpatient illnesses and their care typically occur over more than one visit, often over months or even years, thereby providing lengthy interludes for extensive learning. Just as with inpatient services, the outpatient setting is particularly well suited to role-modeling and interweaving evidence with other topics. The types of rounds that occur in outpatient areas are summarized in Table 7.6; we will focus on the EBM teaching strategies and resources appropriate to each of them.

The "clinic conferences", typically devoted to reviewing the diagnosis and management of common outpatient disorders, can abandon passive annual lectures and devote themselves to reviewing and discussing new evidence that guides key clinical decisions for these conditions, emphasizing the use of pre-appraised or filtered resources. Participants can make new concise summaries of the evidence, or review and update the prior years' versions, then store these summaries nearby for ongoing use in their practices. Active learning occurs, and senior trainees can be asked to help their junior colleagues "learn the ropes" of how to take part in these processes.

Initial outpatient visits share objectives and constraints with "post-take" rounds on new inpatient admissions, so the same strategies apply. These are quick demonstrations of evidence-based bits of the clinical exam and how to get from pre-test to post-test probabilities of the initial diagnosis, plus instantly available (<15 seconds) evidence about key diagnostic and treatment decisions.

Follow-up visits usually occur long enough after initial visits to allow learners to accomplish substantial problem-based learning between visits, that can even be in multiple stages. When the learner first encounters an ambulatory patient, the teacher can coach them on the process of asking an answerable clinical question about one of the patient's problems and writing an educational prescription. At

Table 7.6 Incorporating EBM into outpatient rounds

Type of round	Objectives	Evidence of highest relevance	Restrictions[a]	Strategies
Clinic conference (before or after each half-day session, by small groups of learners and attendees)	Review the diagnosis and management of common outpatient disorders	Manifestations of disease, differential diagnosis, pre-test probability, accuracy and precision of diagnostic tests, efficacy and safety of treatment	Time, tardiness, and duties elsewhere	Educational prescriptions for foreground questions (and fact follow-ups for background questions); use, make or update concise summaries of evidence, such as CATs
Preceptorship during initial visits	Decide on working diagnosis and therapy	Accuracy and precision of clinical exam and diagnostic tests; efficacy and safety of initial therapy	Time, incomplete information	Demonstrate evidence-based exam and getting from pre-test to post-test probability; provide pre-assembled evidence summaries on diagnostic tests and initial treatment; write educational prescriptions
Preceptorship during follow-up visits	Review current status and adjust ongoing therapy	Long-term prognosis; efficacy and safety of alternative treatment options; harms from treatment	Time and changing patient needs	Model incorporation of patients' values (e.g. using LHH); fill educational prescriptions
Ambulatory morning report	Review case of particular outpatient(s)	Anything; most common are diagnostic tests and treatment options	Time; interruptions; widely varying levels of experience	Hold session in room with access to evidence resources; write and fill educational prescriptions; review old and new evidence summaries; give 1-minute summaries on critical appraisal, NNT, etc.

[a]All rounds require confidentiality when discussions of individual patients occur in public areas.

subsequent clinic sessions (and before the patient's follow-up visit) the teacher can review the learner's search strategies and critical appraisal of the evidence found. At the time of patient follow-up, the teacher and the learner can discuss how to integrate the evidence into clinical decisions and actions. The learner can then be asked to write a concise summary of the evidence, which the teacher and learner can review at yet another clinical session. Following up on learning in this way doesn't take long at each stage (usually <5 minutes), yet over time leads to cumulative development of EBM skills.

Finally, some teaching outpatient departments hold "morning reports" similar to those held on the inpatient service. They labor under the same restrictions, but also offer the same variety of opportunities for teaching and learning.

WRITING STRUCTURED SUMMARIES OF EVIDENCE-BASED LEARNING EPISODES

At several points in the above discussion we've mentioned the idea of writing or using a structured summary of evidence to aid our learning. Over the years we've used or heard about several different structures, but the one we find ourselves using most often is the critically appraised topic, or CAT (Table 7.7). A CAT is a structured, one-page summary of the results of an evidence-based learning effort, in which a patient's illness stimulates a learner's question, for which the learner finds evidence, appraises the evidence, and decides whether and how to use that evidence in the care of the patient.[20] Because of its "quick and dirty" nature, a CAT may have limitations. The evidence found and selected for use may not be all there is or even the best there is (thus, a CAT is *not* a systematic review). Because the emphasis is on whether and how to use the evidence in one's own practice setting, the CAT may or may not apply to many or even any other settings (therefore, a CAT is *not* a practice guideline). A CAT might contain errors of calculation or appraisal judgments, and is thus not guaranteed to be error-free or permanent.

Table 7.7 Writing structured summaries of evidence-based learning, or CATs (critically appraised topics)

Why use written summaries or CATs?

1. To summarize and consolidate our learning.

2. To make our learning cumulative, not duplicative.

3. To share our learning efforts with others on our team.

4. To refine our EBM skills.

How should we structure evidence summaries or CATs?

Title: declarative sentence that states the clinical bottom line.

Clinical question: four (or three) components of the foreground question that started it all.

Clinical bottom line: concise statement of best available answer(s) to the question.

Evidence summary: description of methods and/or results in concise form (e.g. table).

Comments: about evidence (e.g. limitations) or how to use it in your own setting.

Citation(s): include evidence appraised and other resources, if appropriate.

Appraiser: so you'll know who did the appraising when you return to it later.

Date CAT was "born"/expiration date: so folks will know when to look again.

Despite these potential limitations, we find writing CATs help us in four ways. First, writing down on one page the question, the answer, and the evidence that supports the answer requires us to summarize the key lesson(s) from an episode of evidence-based learning. Writing a concise summary exercises and disciplines our ability to distill the gist of that learning episode, to *consolidate* our learning, thereby helping us get the most out of it. Second, since many important questions are about common disorders and their management, we can expect to need the knowledge more than once. By storing a CAT for later retrieval, we can make our learning efforts *cumulative* (we start from where we left off last time) rather than *duplicative* (we start all over again). Third, by sharing CATs with others on our clinical team, they can learn from our efforts, too, so learning can multiply. Keep in mind that CATs are most useful to those who make them. Fourth, with repetition and coaching, writing CATs can help us refine our EBM skills.

Rod Jackson has developed some other tools that can facilitate teaching critical appraisal and storage of appraisal summaries. He's made these worksheets (and other useful EBM tools) available on his website (www.epiq.co.nz), and we've provided examples of some of them on the accompanying CD.

INCORPORATING EBM INTO CURRICULA, AND SELECTED EDUCATIONAL EVENTS

Some teachers have the responsibility of planning how to incorporate EBM into the curricula of either undergraduate or graduate medical educational programs, so we'll address some of the considerations in doing this. For those who need more on curricula in general and how to develop, implement and evaluate them, we refer you to other works on these topics.[21–26]

Learners need to learn not only how to practice each EBM step, but also when to do each step and how to integrate EBM with the other tasks of clinical work. In this way, learning EBM resembles learning several other complex "clinical process" skills such as the medical interview and the physical examination. To learn such complex undertakings requires, not only beginning with a good introduction, but also revisiting the field numerous times and building on those experiences that came before. This ideal of "vertical alignment" for curricula in EBM parallels the vertical alignment that others are developing in fields such as mathematics and language arts in grade schools. However, to our knowledge, this ideal has not been fully implemented or evaluated. Short of this ideal, we turn here to considerations involved in introducing EBM into existing educational sessions, illustrated by two common situations: "morning report" and "journal club". Although some issues are specific to these forums, many of the topics will apply to other sessions.

Morning report

In many centers, the individual team's post-call rounds are supplemented by a service-wide conference called "morning report". We've witnessed nearly 50 variations of this conference in our travels, although most share six characteristics: most of the senior residents on the clinical service are present, including chief resident(s); faculty who come often include the program director and/or departmental chair; one (or a few) recent admissions are presented, although they vary in freshness; the cases are selected for their potential educational value; the discussions vary widely, but usually focus on the initial diagnosis and treatment of the presented patients' conditions; and follow-up on prior discussed cases can be presented, with occasional educational extras.[27]

Among a program's existing conferences, morning report has several features that make it uniquely attractive as a place to start integrating EBM into the program's curriculum. Clinical learners present real patients with real illnesses, and then discuss real clinical decisions that need to be made in real-time. If a safe and stimulating learning climate has been established, learners can identify what they already know and what they need to know next in order to make these decisions wisely, yielding many questions that could be asked. Because morning report occurs repeatedly, its multiple sessions allow learning to be multistaged. Also, as evidence and other knowledge are learned and shared among those who attend, the judgments involved in integrating and applying the new knowledge can be explicitly addressed. Given the high visibility of the conference, particularly when it's actively supported by the departmental leadership, learners can see the importance placed on learning clinical medicine in evidence-based ways, and the development of lifelong learning skills. Comparing these features to the list of ten successes in teaching EBM (Table 7.2) shows how much potential success morning report could have.

At the same time, morning report at a given institution may present you with several challenges to incorporating EBM.

First, if those who run morning report have other goals for the session, such as using the time for record-keeping duties, these competing objectives can consume learning time, destroy the learning climate, or derail the learning process altogether. Second, if cases are not presented in a focused way, time can be spent sorting through the clinical data and, if this fails, any learning that occurs may not even fit the patients' illnesses. Third, if the learning climate is unsafe, or if learners' ability to ask questions is reduced, then few of the learners' actual knowledge gaps may get asked as questions. Fourth, teacher or learner inexperience with EBM may lead some participants to retreat to pathophysiologic rationale or personal experience when deciding between test or treatment strategies, rather than risk exposing their rudimentary EBM skills by considering evidence to inform their decisions. Specifically, poor question formulation may lead the group's learning astray, while poor searching may frustrate attempts to find current best evidence, and poor critical appraisal skills may lead to the unwise use of flawed evidence in decisions. Fifth, in some centers, those who attend morning report change very frequently, which confounds attempts to make learning multistaged; thus, how the use of EBM in morning report might require repeated re-orientation, as skills can drift between rotations. Despite these challenges, our own and others' experiences suggest that morning report can become a popular and enduring conference in which to incorporate EBM; we've provided some additional suggestions in Table 7.8.[28,29]

To help you prepare ahead of time to successfully introduce EBM into your morning report, we suggest the following six maneuvers. First, find and cultivate allies who will work with you and advocate for an evidence-based approach to learning in morning report. Some may be in your program, such as chief residents and faculty, while others may be in other disciplines, including librarians, statisticians, clinical pharmacists, and others. Second, negotiate teaching and learning EBM to be part of the goals and methods of morning report, by meeting with or becoming the folks who run the conference at your institution. This may take repeated efforts at persuasion, so keep at them. Third, if

Table 7.8 Developing EBM skills in and out of morning report

EBM skill	During morning report	Elsewhere
Asking questions	In context: cases, decisions Model and see modeled Question drills Practice and feedback	Read materials on how Attend how-to sessions One-on-one coaching See modeled elsewhere
Searching for evidence	Review searches briefly Explain options briefly Invite clinical librarian Refine, not learn anew	Read about searching Attend how-to sessions One-on-one coaching See modeled elsewhere
Critical appraisal	Discuss appraisal briefly Teaching scripts about selected portions Refine, not learn anew	Read about appraisal Attend how-to sessions One-on-one coaching See modeled elsewhere
Integration into decisions	In context: cases, decisions Make judgments explicit Integrate values explicitly Identify factors to weigh	Read about integration Attend how-to sessions One-on-one coaching See modeled elsewhere
Self-evaluation	Model, especially at beginning Use checklists Increase reflection, self- awareness, insight Group feedback	Read about self- evaluation Attend how-to sessions One-on-one coaching See modeled elsewhere

possible, simultaneously negotiate the use of group learning techniques and the development of a healthy learning climate into your morning report, since they are both so important to the success of this effort. Fourth, help assemble the infrastructure needed to learn, practice and teach in evidence-based ways, including quick access to evidence resources and opportunities to learn more about EBM skills outside of morning report. Fifth, prepare some learning materials for EBM, including introductory materials on how to get started, samples of concise evidence summaries, and concise explanations of methods underlying the practice of EBM. Sixth, refine further your own skills in facilitating group discussions and in teaching EBM, whether by getting local coaching or by attending a course in how to teach EBM.

On the first day of the new era, use most of that morning report session to get the group off to a great start, using six tactics. First, identify the main learning goals for your morning report and how EBM fits in; ours' are "to improve our abilities to think through our cases with explicit clinical reasoning and to learn from our cases with evidence-based medicine". Second, have participants assess their current skills for each main learning goal, both globally and then for each skill. Try the "double-you" format: How comfortable do *you* feel with *your* ability to . . .? Don't forget to celebrate learners' courage when they acknowledge they need help. Third, have participants set specific goals for learning EBM in this rotation's morning report, taking care to help them set specific goals that are realistic and focused on their own learning needs. Fourth, negotiate the specific formats you'll use to achieve those learning goals, including issues about the case discussions (e.g. How long and detailed should presentations be? How focused should the discussion be?), about the EBM portions (e.g. How many questions should we aim to formulate? How often should each learner present an educational prescription?), and about how much time you'll spend on each. Fifth, negotiate the ground rules for the group's learning efforts in morning report, including both general issues and any specific to the use of evidence (see suggestions in Table 7.11). Sixth, plan when in the rotation you'll revisit the group's learning objectives and adjust the group's methods; we usually do it both at mid-cycle and at the end of the rotation.

Once your morning report group is up and running, using a combination of case discussions and educational prescriptions (Ch. 1), you may find the following six tactics useful. First, during the case presentations, listen "with both ears" to diagnose both the case and the learner, staying alert to both verbal and non-verbal cues. We use a list of common types of clinical questions (Ch. 1) to help us spot clinical issues and learning needs. Second, help the group select one or a few issues from the case to discuss well, rather than aiming to cover the entire case superficially. This allows the group to pool its knowledge, and find its knowledge gaps, on the way to making sound and explicitly informed decisions. Third, help learners articulate these knowledge gaps as answerable clinical questions, and guide them explicitly in the selection of which questions to pursue. Fourth, as learners report their educational prescriptions, listen carefully to select one (or a very few) teaching point(s) to make about applying this evidence for the decision at hand. Fifth, if needed, be ready to provide a brief (2–5-minute) explanation of one aspect of critical appraisal that has special bearing on the evidence at hand, referring those interested in learning more to sources outside of morning report. Sixth, when debriefing the chief residents after morning report about their teaching skills, include teaching EBM along with the other topics in your coaching.

Journal club

In many clinical centers, journal clubs run like Cheyne–Stokes breathing—alternating a few raspy grunts with prolonged apneic inactivity. Many seem to confuse newness with importance, so on a rotating schedule the participants are asked to summarize the latest issues of pre-assigned journals. This means that the choice of topics is driven, not by patients' or learners' needs, but either by the investors, investigators, and editors who choose which products get studied and which get published, or by the postal workers and web servers who determine which journals get delivered. Little wonder, then, that so many journal clubs are so moribund.

On the other hand, some journal clubs are flourishing, and a growing number of them are explicitly designed and conducted along EBM lines. In the many variations we've run or seen, three different learning goals can be identified: learning about the best evidence to inform clinical decisions, learning about important new evidence that should change our practice, or learning EBM skills. While journal clubs can have more than one learning goal, several of the curricular choices made will depend on which goal is pre-eminent (see Table 7.9). Although departments will vary in the choices they make, many will recognize that taking the "skills-driven" approach first will lead to greater subsequent success with either the "needs-driven" or "evidence-driven" versions.

Table 7.9 Three (potentially competing) goals for evidence-based journal clubs

	"Needs-driven"	"Evidence-driven"	"Skills-driven"
What is the main learning goal?	Learn how best to handle patient problems that are common, serious or vexing	Learn about advances in medical knowledge that should change our practice	Learn the skills for evidence-based practice
What group learning needs are identified?	Group members identify what patient problems they need most help with	Group members identify in what aspects or field they aim to keep current	Group members identify what skills for evidence-based practice they need most to refine
What type of evidence is valued most?	Current best evidence useful for solving problems, of several types (see Table 1.2), even if not brand new or not strong	Recent advances in the field that are valid, important and applicable enough to change our practice (i.e. both new and strong)	Evidence that best allows learners to develop the skills they need, of broad range of types (see Table 1.2), even if not brand new or not strong
Who should select topics and types of evidence?	All participants who share responsibility for solving patient problems	All participants who share responsibility for staying current	Members (usually faculty) responsible for finding learning needs and helping learners develop their skills
Which EBM teaching mode is pre-eminent?	Mode 2 (learning good clinical practice in evidence-based ways)	Mode 2 (developing current awareness in evidence-based ways)	Mode 3 (learning EBM skills)

To help you prepare ahead of time to successfully introduce EBM into your journal club, we suggest the following six maneuvers. First, just as with morning report, find and cultivate the allies, whether from within your department or elsewhere, who will help you achieve your aims. Second, negotiate teaching and learning EBM to be one of the main goals of journal club, again either by meeting with or by becoming those who run the conference. While you're at it, try to negotiate departmental consensus on which of the three learning goals in Table 7.9 will be pre-eminent at your institution. Third, negotiate the use of group learning techniques and the development of a healthy learning climate into your journal club. Fourth, help assemble the infrastructure needed to learn, practice, and teach in evidence-based ways, including quick access to evidence resources and opportunities to learn more about EBM skills outside of journal club. Fifth, prepare some learning materials for EBM, including introductory materials on how to get started, samples of concise evidence summaries, whether your own CATs or from evidence-based pre-appraised sources, and even concise explanations of methods underlying the practice of EBM. Sixth, refine further your own skills in facilitating group discussions and in teaching EBM, whether by getting local coaching or by attending a course on how to teach EBM.

No matter how you balance the learning goals in Table 7.9, each journal club session can be thought of as consisting of three parts:

1. In part 1, journal club members identify some learning needs to be addressed in the future. For a needs-driven group, this can take the form of learners presenting cases where they faced uncertainty in clinical decisions, continuing until there is group consensus that a particular problem (we'll call this "problem C") is worth the time and effort necessary to find its solution. For an evidence-driven group, group members can debate which part of their field they most need to update next (this could be called "field segment C"). For a skills-driven group, the members would discuss and decide which skill for

evidence-based practice they most need to develop or refine (this could then be called "skill C"). No matter which of these three approaches is taken, the group then poses one or more answerable clinical questions (usually foreground ones, as in Ch. 1) with which to start the evidence-based learning episode. Group members then take responsibility (either volunteering or on rotation) for performing a search for evidence to be used—whether the best available for problem C, the newest strong evidence for field segment C, or a useful teaching example for skill C. Groups may have members do this in pairs or triplets, so more experienced members can teach skills to newer folks.

2. In part 2, the results of the evidence search (which we'll label "B") on the previous session's problem, field segment, or skill are shared in the form of photocopies of the abstracts of 4–6 systematic reviews, original articles or other evidence. Club members decide which one or two pieces of evidence are worth studying, and arrangements are made to get copies of the clinical question and evidence to all members well in advance of the next meeting.

3. The main part of the journal club (part 3) is spent in a critical appraisal of the evidence found in response to a clinical question posed two sessions ago and selected for detailed study last session. This segment often begins with the admission that most learners haven't read the articles, so time (6–10 minutes) can be provided for everyone to see if they can determine the validity and clinical applicability of one of the articles, thereby reinforcing rapid critical appraisal. After that interlude, the evidence is critically appraised for its validity, importance, and applicability, and a decision is made about whether and how it could be applied to the patient problems (for needs-driven groups), whether and how it should change current practice (for evidence-driven groups), or whether and how it can build skills for evidence-based practice (for skills-driven groups). Since this is the "pay-off" part of journal club, members may need to be guided to complete parts 1 and 2 quickly enough so there's plenty of time for

part 3. The actual order of these three parts of journal club could be reversed, depending on local circumstances and preferences.

Morning report and journal club illustrate many of the considerations involved when re-orienting existing conferences along evidence-based lines. In Table 7.10, we've gathered our favorite 20 questions to ask when integrating EBM into a conference, grouped into issues of persons, places, times, things, and ideas.

LEARNING MORE ABOUT HOW TO TEACH EBM

As with any complex craft that's built on experience as well as knowledge, becoming excellent at teaching EBM requires extensive deliberate practice. In addition to trying out the strategies and tactics in this chapter, we suggest four additional ideas. First, keep a teaching journal, analogous to a laboratory research notebook, in which you record your observations and interpretations of which teaching methods you've tried, what specifically worked, what specifically you'd like to do better, and what you find in watching others teach and in reading about teaching and learning. Second, look for excellent teachers in your institution who would be willing to observe your teaching and provide individualized feedback and coaching, then work with these mentors to develop your skills. Third, attend one of the growing number of workshops on "How to teach EBM" being held around the world, which provide you with time for deliberate practice and the opportunity to gain useful feedback on your teaching methods. Fourth, because learning in small groups is so much a part of clinical learning and teaching, and because when group learning works well it can powerfully enhance evidence-based learning, we suggest you devote substantial time and effort to refining your skills for learning and teaching in small groups, starting with the material in Table 7.11, and continuing with additional readings.[30–36] Although connected to teaching, the evaluation of learning, practicing, and teaching EBM is so important it deserves its own chapter—and it follows next.

Table 7.10 Twenty questions for integrating EBM into a conference

Persons

1. Who will be the learners, and what are their learning styles and needs?

2. Who will be the teachers, and what are their teaching styles and strengths?

3. Who will need to serve as allies or permission-givers for this to succeed?

4. What conversations and relationships need to be developed for this to succeed?

Places

5. Where will this conference be held?

6. How might the physical space help or hinder learning?

7. How can the physical space be altered to optimize learning?

Times

8. When and for how long will this conference be held?

9. Can the sessions be scheduled to support multiple learning stages?

10. How much time will teachers and learners need to prepare for this conference?

11. How much time will learners need after this conference to receive feedback and to reflect upon, consolidate, clarify, and extend their learning?

12. How much time will teachers need after this conference to give feedback and to reflect upon, cultivate, and refine their teaching?

Things

13. What resources need to be present during the conference?

14. What resources need to be available for teachers and learners before and after the conference?

15. How should participants summarize their evidence-based learning (e.g. CATs or educational prescriptions)?

16. What tools of measurement and evaluation will be used for this conference?

Ideas

17. How well does EBM fit with the other goals of this conference?

18. How can the learning climate be optimized for an evidence-based approach?

19. Which modes of teaching EBM should be emphasized in this conference?

20. How many features of success in teaching EBM (Table 7.2) can be included, while how many mistakes in teaching EBM (Table 7.3) can be avoided?

Table 7.11 Tips for teaching EBM in clinical teams and other small groups[a]

Help team/group members understand why to learn in small groups

Learners may vary in their prior experiences with learning in groups, so they may benefit from reflecting on why it's worth undertaking. Useful points are:

1. Learning in groups allows a broader range of questions about any given topic to be asked and answered, since the work is done by several people. As the results of an individual's effort are shared with others, lessons learned have a "multiplier" effect.

2. Learning in groups allows experienced members to pair with inexperienced members during the work, thereby helping novices to learn faster and reinforcing everyone's capacity for teamwork.

3. The interactive discussions groups use as they learn can help individual members clarify their own misconceptions, consolidate the lessons learned by explaining things to others, and hear multiple viewpoints when considering the implications of the new knowledge for decision and action.

4. Learning in groups allows individual participants to practice performance of skills, using other group members within practice, which helps the individual to learn.

5. Learning in groups also allows individual participants to get feedback on their performance from peers as well as tutors, providing both "reality check" to their own perceptions and suggestions for further learning.

6. The camaraderie, the interpersonal support, and the cohesion from shared challenges and achievements can make learning in groups more fun than learning in isolation.

7. In many fields of work, leaders spend time building groups of individuals into well-functioning work teams, since team performance almost always bests that of individuals.

8. Consider an analogy between group learning and how professional cyclists ride in groups: by riding closely in the peloton to draft and to rotate leading, cyclists can ride faster, longer and farther than even the best of them can ride individually.

Help team/group members set sensible ground rules for small group learning

Small groups can succeed in learning EBM (or anything else) if group members establish effective ways of working together. Useful ground rules include the following:

1. Members take responsibility (individually and as a group) for:

    a. Showing up, and on time.

    b. Learning each other's names, interests and objectives.

    c. Respecting each other.

Table 7.11 *(Cont'd)*

    d. Contributing to, accepting, and supporting individual and group rules of behavior, including confidentiality.

    e. Contributing to, accepting, and supporting both the overall objectives of the group and the detailed plans and assignments for each session.

    f. Carrying out the agreed plans and assignments, including role-playing.

    g. Listening (concentrating and analyzing), rather than simply preparing your own response to what's being said.

    h. Talking (including consolidating and summarizing).

2. Members monitor and (by using time-in/time-out) reinforce positive and correct negative elements of both:

    a. "Process", including:

      • Educational methods (e.g. reinforcing positive contributions and teaching methods; proposing strategies for improving less effective ones).

      • Group functioning (e.g. identifying behaviors, not motives; encouraging non-participants; quieting down over-participators).

    b. "Content", including:

      • Critical appraisal topics (e.g. if unclear, uncertain or incorrect facts or principles, strategies, or tactics about how to carry it out).

      • Clinical matters (e.g. if clinical context or usefulness is unclear).

3. Members evaluate self, each other, the group, the session, and the program with candor and respect:

    a. Celebrating what went well and what should be preserved.

    b. Identifying what went less well, focusing on strategies for correcting or improving the situation.

4. When giving feedback constructively, members do the following:

    a. Give feedback only when asked to do so or when the offer is accepted.

    b. Give feedback as soon after the event as possible.

    c. Focus on the positive; wherever possible give positive feedback first and last.

    d. Be descriptive (of behavior), not evaluative (of motives).

    e. Talk about specific behaviors and give examples where possible.

    f. Use "I" and give your experience of the behavior.

    g. When giving negative feedback, suggest alternative behaviors.

    h. Confine negative feedback to behaviors that can be changed.

Table 7.11 *(Cont'd)*

    i. Ask, "Why am I giving this feedback?" (Is it really to help the person concerned?)

    j. Remember that feedback says a lot about its giver as well as its receiver.

5. When receiving feedback constructively, members do the following:

    a. Listen to it (rather than prepare a response or defense).

    b. Ask for it to be repeated if it wasn't easily heard.

    c. Ask for clarification and examples if statements are unclear or unsupported.

    d. Assume it is constructive until proven otherwise; then, use and consider those elements that are constructive.

    e. Pause and think before responding.

    f. Accept it positively (for consideration) rather than dismissively (for self-protection).

    g. Ask for suggestions of specific ways to modify or change the behavior.

    h. Respect and thank the person giving feedback.

Help team/group members plan the learning activities wisely

During initial introductions, group members should identify their individual learning goals, from which the group can set group learning goals. Tutors and group members should keep these learning goals in mind as they plan the learning objectives for each session, including what to learn, what to emphasize, and how to engage the group in the learning activities. For groups just beginning to learn EBM, consider the following:

1. Plan the session to include a learning situation that is realistic to what group members do in their actual work. For most clinicians, this means using the illnesses of patients actually in their care, or case examples they might encounter frequently.

2. Prepare the question, search and critical appraisal ahead of time, to be familiar with the teaching challenges that may arise. Of the possible questions this case could generate, select one with a high yield in terms of learning, which is usually a mix of the following considerations:

    a. Relevance to the clinical decision being made.

    b. Appropriateness to the learners' prior knowledge.

    c. Availability of good-quality evidence to address the question (so first experience shows positively how evidence can be used once understood and appraised).

    d. Availability of easily understood evidence about the question (so first experience is not too overwhelming methodologically).

    e. Likelihood the question will recur, so learners can benefit more than once.

Table 7.11 *(Cont'd)*

3. As the session begins, engage the group in the clinical situation and have the group focus on the decision to be made. Consider having group members vote on what they would do clinically before the evidence is appraised (if need be, this can be done anonymously).

4. Encourage group members to run the session, yet be prepared to guide them in the early going.

5. As the group works through the critical appraisal portions, emphasize how to understand and use research, rather than how to do research.

6. Summarize important points in the session (if the group is using a scribe, this person could record them for later retrieval).

7. As the session ends, encourage the group to come to closure on how to use the evidence in the clinical decision. Keep in mind that coming to closure needn't require complete agreement; rather, a good airing of the issues that ends in legitimate disagreement can be very instructive.

8. Keep to the time plan overall, but don't worry if the group doesn't cover everything in this one session; if the initial experience goes well, there will be more opportunities.

9. For groups gaining competence and confidence in EBM, the sky is the limit. Encourage the group to invent its own activities, and consider the following:

   a. When selecting questions and evidence to appraise, consider using:

      • Flawed evidence, so the group can develop skill in detecting flaws.

      • A pair of articles, one good and one not so good, for the group to compare.

      • A pair of good articles that reach opposite conclusions.

      • Controversial evidence, so the group learns to disagree constructively.

      • Evidence that debunks current practice, so the group learns to question carefully.

      • A systematic review of early small trials, along with a later definitive trial.

   b. When selecting learning contexts to employ in the group, encourage group members to try out sessions of increasing difficulty, such as practicing teaching jaded senior residents rather than eager students.

   c. When group members disagree, capitalize on the disagreement, by such tactics as:

      • Trying to sort out whether the disagreement is about the data, the critical appraisal, or the values we use in making the judgments.

Table 7.11 *(Cont'd)*

- Framing the disagreement positively, as a chance to understand more deeply.
- Framing the protagonists positively, as providing the group a chance to learn by stating the various perspectives on the topic.
- Wherever possible, keeping the disagreement from becoming personal.

Help team/group members keep a healthy learning climate

The learning climate is the general tone and atmosphere that pervades the group sessions. Encourage the group to cultivate a safe, positive learning climate, wherein group members feel comfortable identifying their limitations and addressing them. Some tactics include the following:

1. Be honest and open about your own limitations and the things you don't know.

2. Model the behavior of turning what you don't know into answerable questions and following through on finding answers, using an educational prescription.

3. Have fun with, and show others the fun in, finding knowledge gaps and learning.

4. Encourage all questions, particularly those that aim for deep understanding.

5. Encourage legitimate disagreement, particularly when handled constructively.

6. Encourage group members to use educational prescriptions.

7. Provide both intellectual challenge (to stimulate learning) and personal support (to help make learning adaptive).

Help team/group members keep the discussion going

1. Early on, model effective facilitating behaviors that encourage discussion, such as:

   a. When someone asks a question, turn the question over to the group and ask them.

   b. If a group member answers another member's question well, ask others in the group for additional effective ways that they've used to answer the same question.

   c. If a group discussion turns into a debate between two members, ask others to provide additional perspective before the group decides.

   d. Don't be afraid of quiet moments, and of using silence when needed.

2. Observe carefully how group members keep discussion moving, and use these observations for feedback and coaching.

Table 7.11 *(Cont'd)*

3. Encourage group members to reflect on what works well in different teaching situations, balancing the desire to move forward with the need to pull everyone along.

Help team/group members keep the discussion on track

1. Early on, model effective facilitating behaviors that help group members to stay focused on the task at hand, such as:

   a. Break the discussion into observable chunks, and set short time for each chunk (e.g. "For the next two minutes, let's brainstorm all the outcomes of clinical interest to us for this condition and its treatment.").

   b. When someone brings up a tangent, identify it non-judgmentally and ask the group how they'd like to handle it.

   c. Reflect to the group what they seem to be discussing, to inform their choices about how to spend their efforts.

2. Observe carefully how group members keep the discussion on track, and use these observations for feedback and coaching.

3. Encourage group members to reflect on what works well for keeping a discussion focused well, while at the same time staying alert for good teaching moments that arise spontaneously.

Help team/group members manage time well

To accomplish their group objectives, group members need to manage their time together effectively. This includes spending time on things that are important and avoiding distractions wherever possible. Some tactics include:

1. At the beginning, model effective time management by encouraging the group to set specific plans for how much time to spend on:

   a. Carrying out the learning activities for the present session.

   b. Evaluating the present session, including giving feedback.

   c. Planning the subsequent session, including revising group objectives.

2. As the group takes charge, coach the members on issues of time management, such as:

   a. How to use a "timekeeper", usually a member not leading that session.

   b. How to adjust time allotted for various functions, after group negotiation.

   c. How to handle new learning issues that arise, which might consume time to address. Here several options exist, including the following:

   - Address it fully right then (if it's important enough and if the group's work would halt without doing so).

Table 7.11 *(Cont'd)*

- Address it briefly at the time, and have a group member (or tutor) address it more completely later, either to the group or with the individual.

- Delay addressing the topic; instead, record it for later discussion (in a place sometimes dubbed the "parking lot").

3. Encourage the group to evaluate time management as the members evaluate the group's functioning.

Help team/group members address some common issues of learning EBM

Jargon

Jargon consists of words from the technical languages of any discipline; for EBM these can be from epidemiology, biostatistics, decision sciences, economics, and other fields. If unexplained, jargon can be intimidating and might delay learning. Some tactics for dealing with jargon include:

1. Introduce and explain the idea first, then label it with the technical term. In this way the understanding comes first, before the word can intimidate.

2. If group members introduce jargon terms, ask them to explain the terms to others in concise ways. This helps the group's understanding, and allows the member to practice brief explanations for later use.

3. Consider having the group keep an accumulating glossary of terms covered, for members to refer to during and after the sessions. You can start with the brief glossary that is in each issue of evidence-based journals such as *ACP Journal Club*.

Quantitative study results

Most reports contain simple calculations, and many contain complex and intimidating ones. Although most of them don't deserve extensive discussion, others, if left unexplained, can needlessly intimidate some learners. Tactics for dealing with quantitative results include:

1. Introduce the concept using real data and work slowly through the arithmetic, so learners can follow the calculations.

2. Use the word names for the arithmetical functions, rather than talking in symbols.

3. Calculate a result from the study data, then introduce its name and a general formula. Just as in dealing with jargon, this order helps demystify the terms.

4. To check their understanding, allow group members time to practice the arithmetic until they feel comfortable enough to move on.

5. Consider having the group keep an accumulating glossary of quantitative results, including names, formulae and uses, for group members to use during and afterwards. Again, the glossaries of EBM journals can provide the nidus for this activity.

Table 7.11 *(Cont'd)*

Statistics

The study's methods and results sections will usually describe the technical devices of statistics used for the research. Some may be familiar to you and your group members, while many may not be. Groups will need to learn how to handle questions about statistics, epidemiology, or any other methodological issue. Some tactics include:

1. Highlight the distinction between statistical and clinical significance, and illustrate with evidence being examined.

2. Assuming the group members want to learn how to understand and use research, rather than do research (worth double-checking now and then), consider advising the group to select a few statistical notions to understand well (e.g. confidence intervals), and point them to resources that can help them (such as the appendix on confidence intervals in this book).

3. Ask the group how deeply they'd like to delve into this topic (many will opt for shallow initial treatment, to allow the group's work to continue, followed by resources for deeper learning later). If they choose deeper amounts, and you cannot provide this on the spot, involve them in choosing among the realistic alternatives, including:

   a. A single group member (or the tutor, if needed) looks up the statistical measure or test and reports back concisely at a later session.

   b. Pairs or small teams from the group find the needed information outside the session, and plan a learning activity around it for a subsequent session.

   c. A nearby statistician is persuaded to join the group temporarily to address the topic at a subsequent session.

4. Remind group members that they may face learners with similar questions upon return home. Coach them in developing answers of different lengths and depths, appropriate for different situations:

   a. "One-liners": for when learners want just enough to get back to other work.

   b. "One-paragraphers": for when learners want more verbal explanation.

   c. "One-siders": one page (or a few) handouts on the topic that might be developed ahead of time, for learners who want a little more depth to read later; this can be coupled with "one-citers" (i.e. a useful citation for even more depth).

5. As the group members run sessions themselves, observe carefully how they handle statistical, epidemiological or other methodological issues and use these observations in coaching and feedback.

6. Ask the group to assess its handling of methodological topics when they evaluate the session.

7. Consider having the group keep a cumulative list of methodological issues covered.

Table 7.11 *(Cont'd)*

Help team/group members identify and deal with counter-productive behaviors

Nihilism

As learners grow in their ability to detect study flaws, some may go through a period of nihilism ("No study is perfect, so what good is any literature?"). Often this occurs in those who can find bias but who don't yet understand its consequences. This negative imbalance is usually temporary, but it can dampen the spirits of others and impede group function. Some tactics are useful in ameliorating this unease:

1. Select good articles at the start, so that early experiences are positive.

2. When using flawed articles, ask the group if something can be learned, even if the study does not provide a definitive answer.

3. Help group members put the study in its knowledge context: What else is known about this? Although potentially flawed, a study may be the earliest in a given field, when the state of prior knowledge is low. Thus, the study may represent incomplete knowledge, rather than bad knowledge.

4. Help group members ask whether missing information is due to poor study design and execution, or to editorial decisions about publishing space. Some data missing in the report may be available from the authors of the study.

5. Help group members separate minor problems from major design flaws that seriously affect the likely validity of results.

6. Help group members ask a series of questions:

   a. Do the study methods allow the possibility of bias?

   b. If so, how much distortion of the results might this bias cause?

   c. If so, in which direction might this bias distort the results?

7. Help group members identify what they would find in an ideal study that answers the question. Then consider how far from ideal is the available evidence.

Discussion tangents

Small group work can stimulate learners, bringing forth not only discussion ideas that would keep the group on their learning spiral, but also discussion ideas that could take the group elsewhere (tangents from the spiral). The energy released can be invigorating, yet, if every topic were to be discussed, the group may not achieve its objectives. Group members need to learn constructive ways of handling possible discussion tangents, some of which are as follows:

1. Identify to the group that a tangent has arisen, validating it as a possibly productive line of learning.

Table 7.11 *(Cont'd)*

2. Ask the group to choose how to proceed, based on their overall learning goals rather than just the plan for that session. This may mean following the tangent, as it might meet their goals better, or it may mean placing the tangent on a list of topics to address later (the "parking lot"). Either way, encourage the group to decide, letting them know you'll stick with them on either path.

3. Some tangents can be turned into extended loops of the learning spiral. That is, these topics can be briefly and concisely discussed, enough to inform the original discussion, to which the group then returns. It may help to set a time limit for such a tangent, and have the timekeeper help the group keep to the limit.

4. When they're running the session, observe closely how group members deal with tangents and use these observations for feedback and coaching.

5. Encourage the group to assess its management of tangents during its evaluation.

A dominating over-participator

Some groups may have one or more members whose personality or enthusiasm leads them to contribute a great deal, perhaps to the point of dominating the time and impeding the group's work and the other members' learning. Some tactics for dealing with this include:

1. Use non-verbal signals (eye contact, hand gestures, body position, etc.) to encourage this person to become quieter and others to contribute more.

2. Seat this person next to one of the tutors, which can encourage moderation.

3. After this person contributes again, ask several others to contribute. This may take reminding the over-participator to let others have a fair turn to speak.

4. Take a time-out to address the group's process, perhaps by reviewing the group's ground rules about participation, or by asking the group to identify the over-participation and make adjustments. In doing so, focus on the behavior (amount and nature of speech), rather than on the person or the motivations for the behavior.

5. Consider suggesting the device of a "peace pipe". This can be any object (originally an actual tobacco pipe used at Native American gatherings) that signifies the person holding it has permission to speak. When finished speaking, that person may give the object to someone else or place it on the table for anyone to choose. This can be a fun and instructive exercise to try, through which group members can discover both under- and over-participation, as well as how many of them talk at once.

Table 7.11 *(Cont'd)*

A quiet non-participator

Some group members are quiet initially, as they "warm up" to the people and the group's activities. Other members may be quiet longer, either from personal style or for other reasons such as language skills. Still others may be quiet due to lack of preparation, for fear of embarrassment, or due to lack of engagement. While not always pathologic, quietness can be a signal to individual or group troubles. Groups will need tactics to recognize and address members who contribute little, some of which are:

1. Be sensitive to reasons for quietness and adjust accordingly. If need be, approach the group member between sessions to find out why.

2. Use non-verbal signals (eye contact, hand gestures, body position, etc.) to encourage this person to contribute more.

3. Seat this person next to one of the tutors, which can encourage participation.

4. Take a time-out to address the group's process, perhaps by reviewing the group's ground rules about participation, or by asking the group to identify the under-participation and make adjustments. In doing so, focus on the behavior (amount and nature of speech), rather than on the person or the motivations for the behavior.

5. Consider pairing the quiet person with another group member for an activity, so they can work together on planning and carrying out this activity. Make sure quiet folks (and all group members) feel more supported as they take on challenges in the group.

6. Consider trying the "peace pipe" (see above). For under-participators, tutors and group members can make it a point to pass it to them, asking them to contribute at least a little before passing it on to others.

Help team/group members prepare for using EBM skills "back home"

As they grow in competence and confidence in their EBM skills, group members will begin to confront how to start or advance their use of EBM in their daily work. For clinicians and teachers, this may mean facing for the first time some of the barriers to incorporating evidence in practice addressed elsewhere in this book. You can help them prepare to overcome these barriers with a mix of enthusiasm, realism, and practicality. Some tactics include:

1. Encourage each group member to select one or a few places to start introducing EBM, rather than trying to start everywhere at once. Consider having them rank three or more candidate activities for introducing EBM, then discussing in buzz groups the advantages and disadvantages of each.

2. Use the group members' collective experience to brainstorm how to prepare to introduce EBM into a given learning activity. This brainstorming might be usefully organized around five areas

Table 7.11 *(Cont'd)*

(persons, places, times, things, and ideas; see Table 7.10) that would need to be considered when introducing EBM "back home".

3. Since changes involving only a few may be easier than changes involving many, it may be wise to work toward an early success by introducing EBM in a way that doesn't require massive shifts in institutional culture. Indeed, the simplest may be a change that involves the actions of only the group member, at least at first. Once momentum is gained, more challenging tasks can be tackled.

4. Encourage group members to be realistic in setting expectations for what can be accomplished early, yet optimistic about what can be achieved in the long-term.

ª Thanks again to Martha Gerrity and Valerie Lawrence, who compiled an early version of this list that was published in this book's first edition. Since then, we've kept changing the list as we've gained more experience with small group learning, and because we can't resist the urge to tinker.

REFERENCES

1 Schon DA. Educating the Reflective Practitioner. San Francisco: Jossey-Bass, 1987.

2 Candy PC. Self-Direction for Lifelong Learning: A Comprehensive Guide to Theory and Practice. San Francisco: Jossey-Bass, 1991.

3 Neighbour R. The Inner Apprentice. Newbury: Petroc Press, 1996.

4 Ericsson KA, ed. The Road to Excellence: The Acquisition of Expert Performance in the Arts and Sciences, Sports and Games. Mahwah: Lawrence Erlbaum, 1996.

5 Davis D, Thomson MA. Continuing medical education as a means of lifelong learning. In: Silagy C, Haines A, eds. Evidence-Based Practice in Primary Care. London: BMJ Books, 1998.

6 Palmer PJ. The Courage to Teach: Exploring the Inner Landscape of a Teacher's Life. San Francisco: Jossey-Bass, 1998.

7 Claxton G. Wise-Up: The Challenge of Lifelong Learning. New York: Bloomsbury, 1999.

8 Davis DA, O'Brien MA, Freemantle NA, et al. Impact of formal continuing medical education: do conferences, workshops, rounds and other traditional continuing education activities change physician behavior or health care outcomes? JAMA 1999; 282: 867–94.

9 Bransford JD, Brown AL, Cocking RR, eds. How People Learn: Brain, Mind, Experience, and School. Washington: National Academy Press, 2000.

10 Brown JS, Duguid P. The Social Life of Information. Boston: Harvard Business School Press, 2000.

11 Davis DA, Barnes B, Fox RD, eds. The Continuing Professional Development of Physicians. Chicago: AMA Press, 2002.

12 Parkes J, Hyde C, Deeks J, Milne R. Teaching critical appraisal skills in health care settings. Cochrane Library, Issue 1. Oxford: Update Software, 2004.

13 Pinsky LE, Monson D, Irby DM. How excellent teachers are made: reflecting on success to improve teaching. Adv Health Sci Educ 1998; 3: 207–15.

14 Dodek PM, Sackett DL, Schechter MT. Systolic and diastolic learning: an analogy to the cardiac cycle. CMAJ 1999; 160: 1475–7.

15 Pinsky LE, Irby DM. If at first you don't success: using failure to improve teaching. Acad Med 1997; 72: 973–6.

16 Smith R. Thoughts for new medical students at a new medical school. BMJ 2003; 327: 1430–3.

17 Ellis J, Mulligan I, Rowe J, Sackett DL. Inpatient general medicine is evidence-based. Lancet 1995; 346: 407–10.

18 Sackett DL, Straus SE. Finding and applying evidence during clinical rounds: the evidence cart. JAMA 1998; 280: 1336–8.

19 Richardson WS, Burdette SD. Practice corner: taking evidence in hand. ACP J Club 2003: 138; A9.

20 Sauve S, Lee HN, Meade MO, Lang JD, Farkouh M, Cook DJ, Sackett DL. The critically appraised topic: a practical approach to learning critical appraisal. Ann R Coll Physicians Surg Canada 1995; 28: 396–8.

21 Hunter KM. Eating the curriculum. Acad Med 1997; 72: 167–72.

22 Kern DE, Thomas PA, Howard DM, Bass EB. Curriculum Development for Medical Education: A Six-Step Approach. Baltimore: Johns Hopkins University Press, 1998.

23 Ornstein AC, Hunkins FP. Curriculum: Foundations, Principles, and Issues, 3rd edn. Boston: Allyn and Bacon, 1998.

24 Green ML. Identifying, appraising, and implementing medical education curricula: a guide for medical educators. Ann Intern Med 2001; 135: 889–96.

25 Kaufman DM. ABC of learning and teaching in medicine: applying educational theory in practice. BMJ 2003; 326: 213–16.

26 Prideaux D. ABC of learning and teaching in medicine: curriculum design. BMJ 2003; 326: 268–70.

27 Amin Z, Guajardo J, Wisniewski W, Bordage G, Tekian A, Niederman LG. Morning report: focus and methods over the past three decades [review]. Acad Med 2000; 75 (10 Suppl): S1–S5.

28 Richardson WS. Teaching evidence-based medicine in morning report. Clin Epidemiol Newsl 1993; 13: 9.

29 Reilly B, Lemon M. Evidence-based morning report: a popular new format in a large teaching hospital. Am J Med 1997; 103: 419–26.

30 Tiberius RG. Small Group Teaching: A Troubleshooting Guide. Toronto: OISE Press, 1990.

31 Jason H, Westberg J. Fostering Learning in Small Groups: A Practical Guide. Philadelphia: Springer, 1996.

32 Brookfield SD, Preskill S. Discussion as a Way of Teaching: Tools and Techniques for Democratic Classrooms. San Francisco: Jossey-Bass, 1999.

33 Maudsley G. Roles and responsibilities of the problem based learning tutor in the undergraduate medical curriculum. BMJ 1999; 318: 657–61.

34 Jaques D. Learning in Groups, 3rd edn. London: Kogan Page, 2000.

35 Wood DF. ABC of learning and teaching in medicine: problem based learning. BMJ 2003; 326: 328–30.

36 Jaques D. ABC of learning and teaching in medicine: teaching small groups. BMJ 2003; 326: 492 4.

Evaluation

The fifth step in practicing EBM is self-evaluation; we'll suggest some approaches for doing that in this final chapter. This book is geared to help individual clinicians to learn how to practice EBM; this section will therefore focus mainly on how we can reflect on our own practice. However, some of us are also involved in teaching EBM, and we've provided some tips on how to evaluate our teaching; additional relevant material is available on the accompanying CD. And, some clinicians, managers, and policy-makers might be interested in evaluating how EBM is being implemented at a local, regional, or national level; although this is not the aim of this book, we'll point you to some useful resources.

HOW AM I DOING?

As you might have guessed by now, we believe that the most important evaluations of our performance are the ones we design and carry out ourselves. Accordingly, this part of the chapter will describe the domains in which you might want to evaluate your performance. We also will note some aids to self-evaluation that you can find on the book's CD.

Evaluating our performance in asking answerable questions

We'd suggest asking ourselves five questions (Table 8.1). These questions are about our own question-asking in practicing EBM. First, are we asking any questions at all? And, as we begin to do so, are they well formulated? As our experience grows, are we using a map of where most questions come from (Table 1.2 is our version) to locate our knowledge gaps, and help us articulate questions? When we get stuck, are we increasingly able to get "unstuck" using the map or other devices? On a practical level, have we devised a method to note our questions as they occur, for later retrieval and answering when time permits? There are

8

Table 8.1 Self-evaluation in asking answerable questions

1. Am I asking any clinical questions at all?

2. Am I asking well-formulated questions:

   • Two-part questions about "background" knowledge?

   • Four- (or three-) part questions about "foreground" diagnosis, management, etc.?

3. Am I using a "map" to locate my knowledge gaps and articulate questions?

4. Can I get myself "unstuck" when asking questions?

5. Do I have a working method to save my questions for later answering?

---

low-tech and high-tech options for this; some of us keep a logbook in our pocket to record our questions and the answers when we've had a chance to retrieve them. Alternatively, we could go for the high-tech option and use a program that we've devised for PDAs (available on the CD) which allows us to record our questions and answers.

Evaluating our performance in searching

Table 8.2 lists some questions we might want to ask ourselves about our performance in searching for the best external evidence. Again, are we searching at all? Do we know the best sources of current evidence for our clinical discipline? Are we trying to find the highest quality evidence, aiming for the top of the "information pyramid" (Figure 2.1) as described in Chapter 2? Have we achieved immediate access to searching hardware, software, and the best evidence for our clinical discipline? Are the most crucial resources bookmarked? You might wish to try timing the steps in your search process: locating a resource, starting up the resource, typing in a question, getting the response, etc. Which of these can you speed up to become more efficient with this process? If we have started searching on our own, are we finding useful external evidence from a widening array of sources, and are we becoming more efficient in our searching? Are we

Table 8.2 A self-evaluation in finding the best external evidence

1. Am I searching at all?

2. Do I know the best sources of current evidence for my clinical discipline?

3. Have I achieved immediate access to searching hardware, software, and the best evidence for my clinical discipline?

4. Am I finding useful external evidence from a widening array of sources?

5. Am I becoming more efficient in my searching?

6. Am I using truncations, booleans, MeSH headings, thesaurus, limiters, and intelligent free text when searching MEDLINE?

7. How do my searches compare with those of research librarians or other respected colleagues who have a passion for providing best current patient care?

using MeSH headings, thesaurus, limiters, and intelligent free text when searching MEDLINE? Are we using validated search filters when using MEDLINE?

An efficient way of evaluating our searching skills is to ask research librarians or other respected colleagues to repeat a search that we've already done and then compare notes on both the searching strategy and the usefulness of the evidence we both found. Done this way, we benefit in three ways: from the evaluation itself, from the opportunity to learn how to do it better, and from the yield of additional external evidence on the clinical question that prompted our search.

It might be wise to consult our nearest health sciences library about taking a course or personal tutorial, so that we can get to the level of expertise we need to carry out this second step in practicing EBM. We might even persuade one of the librarians to join our clinical team—an extraordinary way to increase our proficiency!

Evaluating our performance in critical appraisal
Table 8.3 lists some questions to examine how we're doing in critically appraising external evidence. Are we doing it at all?

> **Table 8.3** A self-evaluation in critically appraising the evidence for its validity and potential usefulness
>
> 1. Am I critically appraising external evidence at all?
> 2. Are the critical appraisal guides becoming easier for me to apply?
> 3. Am I becoming more accurate and efficient in applying some of the critical appraisal measures (such as likelihood ratios, NNTs, and the like)?
> 4. Am I creating any appraisal summaries?

If not, can we identify the barriers to our performance and remove them? Once again, we might find that working as a member of a group (such as the different sort of journal club we describe in Ch. 7) could not only help us get going but also give us feedback about our performance.

Most clinicians find that critical appraisal of most types of articles becomes easier with time, but find one or two that continue to confuse. Again, this is a situation in which working in a group (even "virtual" groups) can quickly identify and resolve such confusion. We can then proceed to consider whether we are becoming more accurate and efficient in applying some of the measures of effect (such as likelihood ratios, NNTs and the like). This could be done by comparing our results with those of colleagues who are appraising the same evidence, or by taking the raw data from an article abstracted in one of the journals of secondary publication, completing the calculations, and then comparing them with the abstract's conclusions.

Finally, at the most advanced level, are we creating summaries of our appraisals? We could use formal CATMaker software to create these summaries, or we could develop our own template for storing appraisals. We find CATMaker a useful teaching tool, but often we find it too cumbersome for use in our clinical practice; instead, we keep abbreviated versions of our appraisals using a simple template, which includes the study citation, clinical bottom line, a two-line description of the study methods, and a brief table or summary of results.

Evaluating our performance in integrating evidence and patients' values

Table 8.4 lists some elements of a self-evaluation of our skills in integrating our critical appraisals with our clinical expertise and applying the results in our clinical practice. Not surprisingly, it opens by suggesting that we ask ourselves whether we are integrating our critical appraisals into our practice at all. Because the efforts we've expended in the previous three steps are largely wasted if we can't execute this fourth one, we'd need to do some soul-searching and carry out some major adjustments of how we spend our time and energy if we're not following through on it. Once again, talking with a mentor or working as a member of a group might help overcome this failure, as might attending one of the EBM workshops. Once we are on track, we could ask ourselves whether we are becoming more accurate and efficient in adjusting some of the critical appraisal measures to fit our individual patients. Have we been able to find or otherwise establish pre-test probabilities that are appropriate to our patients and the disorders we commonly seek in them?

Are we becoming more adept at modifying measures such as the NNT (number needed to treat) to take into account the "f" for our patient? One way to test our growing skills in this integration is to see whether we can use them to explain (and maybe even resolve!) disagreements about management decisions. We can do this amongst our colleagues in our practice or our residents on the teaching service.

Table 8.4 A self-evaluation in integrating the critical appraisal with clinical expertise and applying the result in clinical practice

1. Am I integrating my critical appraisals into my practice at all?

2. Am I becoming more accurate and efficient in adjusting some of the critical appraisal measures to fit my individual patients (pre-test probabilities, NNT/f, etc.)?

3. Can I explain (and resolve) disagreements about management decisions in terms of this integration?

Is our practice improving?

Although a self-evaluation showing success at the foregoing level should bring enormous satisfaction and pride to any clinician, we might want to proceed even further, and could ask ourselves whether what we have learned has been translated into better clinical practice (Table 8.5). A useful tool to look at this is the plan–do–check–act cycle developed for quality improvement (Figure 8.1 shows a version adapted for use with EBM). The "plan" phase begins with the four steps of question, search, appraise, and apply. It also requires that we consider any barriers to implied changes in our practice. Do we need new skills, equipment, organizational

---

Table 8.5 A self-evaluation of changing practice behavior

1. When new evidence suggests a change in practice, am I identifying barriers to this change?
2. Have I carried out any check, such as audits of my diagnostic, therapeutic, or other EBM performance?

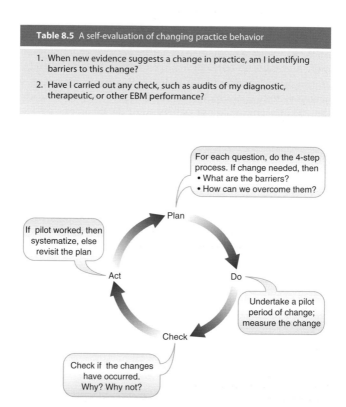

For each question, do the 4-step process. If change needed, then
• What are the barriers?
• How can we overcome them?

If pilot worked, then systematize, else revisit the plan

Undertake a pilot period of change; measure the change

Check if the changes have occurred. Why? Why not?

Figure 8.1 The plan–do–check–act cycle for evaluating how we practice EBM.

processes or a reminder system to prevent memory slips? For example, in one of our practices, we decided that diabetic patients should get annual foot checks, including monofilament testing. To implement this, we needed the monofilaments, the skills to use them reliably, and a data entry field added to our annual check-up form as a reminder to test; the result was a 50% reduction in unnecessary podiatry referrals.

Having planned what to "do", we need to do it. And, once we implement the change, we might wish to "check" that changes have actually occurred (and sometimes we get surprises!) Checks can include audits of our clinical practice, which can be important for two reasons. First, they can tell us how we are performing as clinicians. Second, and far more important, they often incorporate strategies, especially individualized feedback, that can have a very positive effect on our clinical performance. (While we don't reckon that this is a reason to complete an audit, a bonus for completion is that many professional organizations provide CME— continuing medical education—credits for conducting them.)

Audits can occur at various levels of complexity, and many hospitals have well-developed audit (or quality improvement) committees with full-time staff. Because this book is directed to individual clinicians, we won't devote space to audits carried out at these higher levels of organization.* Rather, we'll focus on audits that can be accomplished by individual clinicians and their teams. Practice audits are often carried out at a local, regional or national level, and attempts focused on how to change physician behavior at these levels. Several methods have been found to be effective, including academic detailing, opinion leaders, and electronic reminders. As we've mentioned before, this is not the focus of this book and we refer you to a recent book edited by Dave Davis and colleagues† on this topic.

---

* Gray M. Evidence-based Health Care. Edinburgh: Churchill Livingstone, 1997.

† Davis D, Barnes B, Fox F, eds. The Continuing Professional Development of Physicians: From Research to Practice. Chicago: American Medical Association, 2003.

If the audit shows that we've changed, then we can celebrate and then perhaps consider how to improve further. If we haven't changed, rather than self-recriminations, we should ask what were the problems and barriers to change. And thus we re-enter the cycle with a new plan.

How much of our practice is evidence-based?

A number of clinical teams have looked at the extent to which practice is evidence-based. The impetus for their work was the "conventional wisdom" that only about 20% of clinical care was based in solid scientific evidence.* One of the first studies was performed on David Sackett's clinical service in Oxford, where, at the time of their discharge, death, or retention in hospital at the end of the audited month, every patient was discussed at a team meeting and consensus reached on their primary diagnosis (the disease, syndrome, or condition that was entirely or, in the case of multiple diagnoses, most responsible for the patient's admission to hospital) and their primary intervention (the treatment or other maneuver that represented the most important attempt to cure, alleviate, or care for the primary diagnosis). The primary intervention was then traced, either into an "instant resource book of evidence-based medicine" maintained by the consultant, or to other sources (medical texts, or, via computerized bibliographic database searching, into the published literature), and classified into one of three categories: interventions whose value (or non-value) is established in one or more randomized controlled trials or, better yet, systematic reviews of RCTs (randomized controlled trials); interventions whose face-validity is so great that randomized trials assessing their value were unanimously judged by the team to be both unnecessary and, if they involved placebo treatments, unethical; and interventions in common use but failing to meet either of the preceding two criteria. Of the 109 patients diagnosed that month, 90 (82%) were judged by pre-set criteria to have received evidence-based interventions. The primary

---

* 1963, the estimate was 9.3%. Med Care 1963; 1: 10–6.

interventions for 53% of patients were based on one or more randomized trials or systematic reviews of trials. An additional 29% of patients received interventions unanimously judged to be based on convincing non-experimental evidence, and 18% received specific symptomatic and supportive care without substantial evidence that it was superior to some other intervention or to no intervention at all.

This audit confirmed that inpatient general medicine could be evidence-based, and similar audits since then have been conducted in various settings around the world and in many different clinical disciplines, including general surgery, hematology, child health, primary care, anesthesia and psychiatry. The truth is that most patients we encounter have one of just a few common problems, while the rare problems are thinly spread between many patients. As a result, searching for the evidence that underpins the common problems provides a greater and more useful reward for our effort than fruitless quests for evidence about problems we might encounter once a decade. That these studies have found evidence for the most common interventions has validated the feasibility of practicing EBM. The key point for readers of this book is to recognize how such audits not only focus on clinical issues that are central to providing high-quality evidence-based care but also provide a natural focus for day-to-day education, helping every member of the team keep up-to-date.

Evaluating our performance as teachers

We may be interested in evaluating our own EBM teaching skills or in evaluating an EBM workshop, or course. Table 8.6 lists some ways of evaluating how we're doing as teachers of EBM. When did we last issue an educational prescription (or have one issued to us)? If not, why not? Are we helping our trainees learn how to ask answerable (four-part) questions? Are we teaching and modeling searching skills? Our time may be far too limited to provide this training ourselves, but we should be able to find some help for our learners, and we should try to link them with our local librarians (again, if a librarian can join

Table 8.6 A self-evaluation in teaching EBM
1. When did I last issue an educational prescription?
2. Am I helping my trainees learn how to ask answerable (four-part) questions?
3. Are we incorporating question asking and answering into everyday activities?
4. Are my learners writing educational prescriptions for me?
5. Am I teaching and modeling searching skills (or making sure that my trainees learn them)?
6. Am I teaching and modeling critical appraisal skills?
7. Am I teaching and modeling the generation of appraisal summaries?
8. Am I teaching and modeling the integration of best evidence with my clinical expertise and my patients' preferences?
9. Am I developing new ways of evaluating the effectiveness of my teaching?
10. Am I developing new EBM educational material?

our clinical team, we can share the teaching). Are we teaching and modeling critical appraisal skills, and teaching and modeling the generation of appraisal summaries? Are we teaching and modeling the integration of best evidence with our clinical expertise and our patients' preferences? Are we developing new ways of evaluating the effectiveness of our teaching? Particularly important here are the development and use of strategies for obtaining feedback from our students and trainees about our skills and performance in practicing and modeling EBM. Finally, are we developing new EBM educational materials?

A very useful way of evaluating our performance is to ask our respected colleagues and mentors for feedback. We can invite our colleagues to join our clinical team or to view a video of our teaching performance and to discuss it with us afterward, giving us and them a chance to learn together. We might also seek out a workshop on EBM to refine our skills further.

EVALUATIONS OF STRATEGIES FOR TEACHING THE STEPS OF EBM

Professional organizations and medical schools have moved from whether to teach EBM to how to teach EBM. We therefore might be interested in evaluating how EBM is taught in a course or at a workshop. The next section will summarize evidence on strategies for teaching the elements of EBM. We'll use the "PICO" format ("patients", "intervention", "control maneuver", "outcomes") for our discussion.

Who are the "patients"?

Who are the targets for our clinical questions? Two groups can be readily identified: the clinicians who practice EBM, and the patients they care for. There is an accumulating body of evidence relating to the impact of EBM on students and health care professionals. This ranges from systematic reviews of training in the skills of EBM to qualitative research describing the experience of EBM practitioners and barriers they've encountered to implementation. There is a paucity of evidence about the effect of EBM on patient care or patients' perceptions of their care, but we are starting to see these outcomes being considered.

What is the intervention (and the control maneuver)?

Studies of the effect of teaching EBM are challenging to conduct because, not only would they require large sample sizes and lengthy follow-up periods, but it's unethical to generate a comparison group of clinicians who'd be allowed to become out-of-date and ignorant of life-saving evidence accessible to and known by the evidence-based clinicians in the experimental group. Similarly, it would be tough to get clinicians to agree to an evidence-poor teaching intervention!

In many studies of the impact of EBM, the intervention has proven difficult to define. It's unclear what the appropriate "dose" or "formulation" should be. Some studies use an approach to clinical practice, while others use training in one of the discrete "microskills" of EBM such as MEDLINE searching or critical appraisal. Indeed, a recent review of graduate medical education in EBM found 18 reports of such curricula, but the courses most commonly focused on critical appraisal skills, in many cases to the exclusion of other EBM skills.[1] And, some studies looked at 90-minute workshops, whereas others included courses that were held over several weeks to months. Although the introduction of EBM into undergraduate and postgraduate learning is underway, the challenge is to precede these changes with solid evidence that they will work. And, although this challenge has rarely been set or met by previous architects of new curricula, we nonetheless have sought it here.

What are the relevant outcomes?

Effective EBM interventions will produce a wide range of outcomes. Changes in clinicians' knowledge and skills are relatively easy to detect and demonstrate. Changes in their behaviors and attitudes are harder to confirm. And, as mentioned previously, changes in clinical outcomes are even more challenging to detect. Accordingly, studies demonstrating better patient survival when practice is evidence-based (and worse when it is not) are at present limited to the cohort "outcomes research" studies described in this book's Introduction.

As discussed above, the intervention has proven difficult to define and, as a result, the evaluation of whether the intervention has met its goals has been challenging. In the Introduction we outlined that not all clinicians want or need to learn how to practice all five steps of EBM. We discussed three potential methods for practicing EBM, including the doing, using, and replicating modes. "Doers" of EBM practice steps 1–5, while "users" focus on searching for and applying pre-appraised evidence. "Replicators" seek advice from colleagues who practice EBM. While all of us practice in these different modes at various times in our clinical work, our activity will likely fall predominantly into one of these categories. Most clinicians consider themselves users of EBM, and surveys of clinicians show that only approximately 5%

believe that learning the five steps of EBM was the most appropriate method for moving from opinion-based to evidence-based medicine.[2] The various EBM courses, workshops, and the like must therefore address the needs of these different learners. One size cannot fit all! And similarly, if a formal evaluation of the educational activity is required, the instruments used to evaluate whether we've helped our learners reach their goals should reflect the different learners and their goals. While there have been many questionnaires that have been shown to be useful in assessing EBM knowledge and skills, we must remember that the learners, knowledge, and skills targeted by these tools may not be similar to our own.*

It should be noted that quite innovative methods of evaluation are being used as attention is moving from assessing not just EBM knowledge and skills but to behaviors, attitudes, and clinical outcomes as well. For example, in a study evaluating an EBM curriculum in a family medicine training program, resident–patient interactions were videotaped and analyzed for EBM content.[3] And, EBM-OSCE stations have become standard in many medical schools and residency programs. Finally, some studies currently underway are measuring clinical outcomes.

1. Effects of teaching strategies on searching skills

Several studies have shown that we can improve searching skills. A randomized trial among first clinical year medical students in Oxford showed that a 3-hour session on question formulation and database-searching produced significant gains in the quality of evidence retrieved.[4] The failure of control students to gain these skills by "diffusion" means that these skills must be formally learnt. Similar improvements in searching MEDLINE, sustainable at up to

---

* For those interested in further discussion of the evaluation of EBM, we invite you to take a look at our website where we provide details about groups who are involved with various activities in this field, such as the SGIM-EBM Task Force which is creating a clearing- house of EBM evaluation items, including details about their measurement characteristics.

9 months of follow-up, have been found in postgraduate training programs.[5]

2. Effects of teaching strategies on critical appraisal skills

A review of seven studies that evaluated courses teaching critical appraisal skills showed gains in knowledge (as assessed by a written test) by undergraduates.[6] Postgraduates showed a smaller change in knowledge following a critical appraisal course. A more recent Cochrane Review found only one study that met the authors' inclusion criteria.[7] This study (n = 44) found that a critical appraisal course increased knowledge of critical appraisal in the intervention group compared to the control group. No studies have found that such courses lead to an increase in use of medical literature or in time spent reading.

3. Effects of teaching strategies on clinical decision-making

An undergraduate program adopting problem-based, self-directed learning around diagnosis and therapy has been shown to result in clerks making more and better clinical decisions, which they are better able to defend than peers educated in a more conventional program.[8] Graduates of a problem-based medical school were found to be more up-to-date in the knowledge of the management of hypertension than graduates of a traditional curriculum.[9] In a before-and-after study, a multicomponent EBM intervention including teaching EBM skills and provision of electronic resources to consultants and house officers at a district general hospital found that the intervention significantly improved evidence-based practice patterns.[10] And, a recent Cochrane Review found that traditional, didactic CME does not lead to changes in clinical behavior.[11] In contrast, active, learner-centered approaches were found to be more effective.

Reports describing evidence-based rejuvenations of traditional educational events are burgeoning, and case reports and a survey of US residency programs have concluded that the determinants of continuing high attendance at postgraduate journal clubs are mandatory attendance, the teaching of critical appraisal skills, emphasizing the primary literature, independence from faculty, and (of course) free food![12,13] Finally, qualitative research has confirmed that teaching and learning critical appraisal are enjoyable, a fact that should not be underestimated in one's working life!

For those of you who have read this far, that's it, we're done! We hope you have enjoyed this book and its accompanying resources, as well as learned from them; we would appreciate your suggestions on how to make them more useful as well as more enjoyable.

Cheers.

REFERENCES

1 Green ML. Graduate medical education training in clinical epidemiology, critical appraisal and evidence-based medicine: a critical review of curricula. Acad Med 1999; 74: 686–94.

2 McColl A, Smith H, White P, Field J. General practitioner's perceptions of the route to evidence-based medicine: a questionnaire survey. BMJ 1998; 315: 361–5.

3 Ross R, Verdieck A. Introducing an evidence-based medicine curriculum into a family practice residency: is it effective? Acad Med 2003; 78: 412–17.

4 Rosenberg W, Deeks J, Lusher A, et al. Improving searching skills and evidence retrieval. J R Coll Physicians London 1998; 328: 557–63.

5 Smith CA, Ganschow P, Reilly BM, et al. Teaching residents evidence-based medicine skills. J Gen Intern Med 2000; 15: 710–15.

6 Norman G, Shannon SI. Effectiveness of instruction in critical appraisal skills: a critical appraisal. CMAJ 1998; 158: 177–81.

7 Parkes J, Hyde C, Deeks J, Milne R. Teaching critical appraisal skills in health care settings. Cochrane Library, Issue 4. Oxford: Update Software, 2003 (review updated 2001).

8 Bennett K, Sackett DL, Haynes RB, et al. A controlled trial of teaching critical appraisal of the clinical literature to medical students. JAMA 1987; 257: 2451–4.

9 Shin JH, Haynes RB, Johnston M. Effect of problem-based, self-directed undergraduate education on lifelong learning. CMAJ 1993; 148: 969–76.

10 Straus SE, Ball C, McAlister FA, et al. Teaching evidence-based medicine skills can change practice in a community hospital. (under review)

11 Thomson O'Brien MA, Freemantle N, Oxman A, et al. Continuing education meetings and workshops: effect on professional practice and health care outcomes. Cochrane Library, Issue 4. Oxford: Update Software, 2003 (review updated 2000).

12 Sidorov J. How are internal medicine residency journal clubs organized and what makes them successful? Arch Intern Med 1995; 155: 1193–7.

13 Alguire PC. A review of journal clubs in postgraduate medical education. J Gen Intern Med 1998; 13: 347–53.

Appendix 1: Confidence intervals*

STATISTICAL INFERENCE

What does the "confidence interval" (CI) tell us? The CI gives a measure of the precision (or uncertainty) of study results for making inferences about the population of all such patients. A strictly correct definition of a 95% CI is that 95% of such intervals will contain the true population value. Little is lost by the less pure interpretation of the CI as "a range of values within which we can be 95% sure that the true value lies". Use of the CI places a clear emphasis on quantification of effect, in direct contrast to the P values, which arise from the significance testing approach. The P value is not an estimate of any quantity but rather a measure of the strength of evidence against the null hypothesis of "no effect". The P value by itself tells us nothing about the size of a difference, nor even the direction of that difference. P values on their own are thus not informative in papers or abstracts. By contrast, CIs indicate both quantities of direct interest, such as treatment benefit, and also the strength of the evidence.[1–3] They are thus of particular relevance to practitioners of evidence-based medicine (EBM).

The estimation approach to statistical analysis exemplified in the CI aims to quantify the effect of interest (the sensitivity of a diagnostic test, the rate of a prognostic event, the relative risk reduction for a treatment, etc.), as well as to quantify the uncertainty in this effect. Most often the CI is a range of values either side of the estimate in which we can be 95% sure that the true value lies. The convention of using the value of 95% is arbitrary, just as is that of taking P<0.05 as being statistically significant, and authors sometimes use 90% or 99% CIs. Note that the word "interval" means a range of

* Prepared for this book by Douglas G Altman of the Cancer Research UK Medical Statistics Group, and the Centre for Statistics in Medicine, Oxford, UK

values and is thus singular. The two values that define the interval are called "confidence limits".

The CI is based on the idea that the same study carried out on different samples of patients would not yield identical results, but that their results would be spread around the true but unknown value. The CI estimates this "sampling variation". The CI does *not* reflect additional uncertainty due to other causes; in particular CIs do not incorporate the impact of selective loss to follow-up, poor compliance with treatment, imprecise outcome measurements, lack of blinding, and so on. CIs thus always underestimate the total amount of uncertainty.

CALCULATING CONFIDENCE INTERVALS

Usually the CI is calculated from the observed estimate of the quantity of interest, such as the difference (d) between two proportions, and the standard error (SE) of the estimate for this difference. An approximate 95% CI is obtained here as $d \pm 1.96$ SE. (The formula will vary according to the nature of the outcome measure and the coverage of the CI.) For example, in a randomized placebo-controlled trial of acellular pertussis vaccine,[4] 72/1670 (4.3%) infants developed pertussis among those receiving the vaccine and 240/1665 (14.4%) did so among the control group. The difference in percentages, known as the absolute risk reduction, is 10.1%. The SE of this difference is 0.99%, so that the 95% CI is $10.1\% \pm 1.96 \times 0.99\%$, and therefore runs from 8.2 to 12.0.

Despite the considerably different philosophical approaches, CIs and significance tests are closely related mathematically. Thus a "significant" P value of $P<0.05$ will correspond to a 95% CI which excludes the value indicating no difference; for example, this value is 0 for the difference between two means or proportions and 1 for a relative risk or odds ratio. (The equivalence of the two approaches may not be exact in a few circumstances.) The prevailing view is that estimation, including CIs, is the preferable approach to summarizing the results of a study, but CIs and P values are complementary and many papers present both.

The uncertainty (imprecision) expressed by a CI is to a large extent related to the square root of the sample size. Small samples provide less information than large ones, and the CI is correspondingly wider in a smaller sample. For example, a paper comparing the characteristics of three tests to diagnose *Helicobacter pylori*[5] reported the sensitivity of the [^{14}C]urea breath test as 95.8% (95% CI, 75 to 100). While the figure of 95.8% is impressive, the small sample of 24 adults with *H. pylori* means that there is considerable uncertainty in that estimate, as shown by the wide CI (the lower limit of 75% represents much poorer performance than the estimate of 95.8%). If the same sensitivity had been observed in a sample of 240, the 95% CI would have been 92.5 to 98.0, allowing much greater confidence that the test has high sensitivity.

In randomized controlled trials (RCTs), non-significant results (i.e. those with P>0.05) are especially prone to misinterpretation. CIs are especially useful here as they show whether the data are compatible with clinically useful true effects. For example, in a randomized trial to compare suturing and stapling for large-bowel anastomosis,[6] wound infection occurred in 10.9% and 13.5% of cases respectively (P = 0.30). The 95% CI for this difference of 2.6% is −2 to +8. Even in this study of 652 patients there thus remains the possibility that there is a modest difference in wound infection rates for the two procedures. In a smaller study, uncertainty is greater. Sung et al[7] carried out a randomized trial to compare octreotide infusion and emergency sclerotherapy for acute variceal hemorrhage in 100 patients. The observed rates of controlled bleeding were 84% in the octreotide group and 90% in the sclerotherapy group, giving P = 0.56. Note that the figures for uncontrolled bleeding are similar to those for wound infection in the study just considered. In this case, however, the 95% CI for the treatment difference of 6% is −7 to +19. This interval is very wide in relation to the 5% difference that was of interest. It is clear that the study cannot rule out a large difference in effectiveness, so that the authors' conclusion that "octreotide infusion and sclerotherapy are equally effective in controlling variceal haemorrhage" is certainly not valid. When, as here, the 95% CI for the absolute risk reduction (ARR) spans zero,

265

the CI for the NNT (number needed to treat) is rather peculiar. The NNT and its CI are obtained by taking reciprocals of the ARR values (and multiplying by 100 when those values are given as percentages). Here we get NNT = 100/6 = 16.6, with 95% CI of −14.3 to 5.3. As noted in footnote "d" of Table A1.1, this CI represents values of NNT from 5.3 to infinity and NNH (number needed to harm) from 14.3 to infinity.

CIs can be constructed for most common statistical estimates or comparisons.[8] For RCTs, these include differences between means or proportions, relative risks, odds ratios, and the NNT.[9] Likewise, CIs can be obtained for all the main estimates arising in studies of diagnosis—sensitivity, specificity, positive predictive value (all of which are simple proportions), and likelihood ratios—and estimates derived from meta-analyses and case–control studies. A computer program for personal computers that covers many of these methods is available with the second edition of *Statistics with Confidence*.[8] Macros for calculating CIs for proportions are available for Excel, SPSS, and Minitab at http://www.uwcm.ac.uk/study/medicine/epidemiology_statistics/research/statistics/proportions.htm.

MULTIPLE ESTIMATES OF TREATMENT EFFECT

While CIs are desirable for the primary results of a study, they are not needed for all results. Further, it is important that the CIs relate to the contrast of clinical interest. For example, when comparing two groups, the appropriate CI is that for the difference between the groups, as illustrated in the above examples, not the individual group CIs. Not only is it unhelpful to give separate CIs for the estimates in each group, this presentation can be quite misleading. Similarly, for a comparison of the treatment effect in different subgroups, the correct approach is to compare the two (or more) estimates directly. It is not valid to suggest that a treatment effect is present in only one subgroup when one CI excludes the value indicating no effect and the other does not.[10] CIs are also helpful when considering results in multiple subgroups. Figure A1.1 shows relative risks of

Table A1.1 Standard errors (SEs) and confidence intervals (CIs) for some clinical measures of interest

Clinical measure	Standard error (SE)	Typical calculation of SE and CI[a]
I. THERAPEUTIC STUDIES		
(a) Outcome is an event—one group		
In general, r events are observed among n patients, so the observed proportion is $p = r/n$. In the illustrative example, $p = 24/60 = 0.4$ (or 40%).		
Proportion (event rate in one group)[b]	$SE = \sqrt{\dfrac{p \times (1-p)}{n}}$ where p is proportion and n is number of patients	If $p = 24/60 = 0.4$ (or 40%): $SE = \sqrt{\dfrac{0.4 \times 0.6}{60}} = 0.063$ (or 6.3%) 95% CI is $40\% \pm 1.96 \times 6.3\%$ or 27.6 to 52.4%[b]
(b) Outcome is an event—comparison of two groups[c]		
In general, r_1 and r_2 events are observed among n_1 and n_2 patients in two groups, so the observed proportions are $p_1 = r_1/n_1$ and $p_2 = r_2/n_2$. In the illustrative example, $p_1 = 15/125$ (or 12%) and $p_2 = 30/120 = 0.25$ (or 25%).[d]		
Absolute risk reduction (ARR)	$SE = \sqrt{\dfrac{p_1(1-p_1)}{n_1} + \dfrac{p_2(1-p_2)}{n_2}}$	$ARR = p_2 - p_1 = 0.13$ (or 13%): $SE = \sqrt{\dfrac{0.12 \times 0.88}{125} + \dfrac{0.25 \times 0.75}{120}} = 0.049$ (or 4.9%) 95% CI is $13\% \pm 1.96 \times 4.9\%$, i.e. 3.4% to 22.6%[b]

Table A1-1 *(Cont'd)*

Clinical measure	Standard error (SE)	Typical calculation of SE and CI[a]
Number needed to treat (NNT)	Not calculated	NNT = 100/ARR = 100/13 = 7.7; CI is obtained as reciprocal of CI for ARR, so 95% CI is 100/22.6 to 100/3.4 or 4.4 to 29.4[e]
Relative risk (RR)	$RR = p_1/p_2$ SE of $\log_e RR = \sqrt{\dfrac{1}{r_1} + \dfrac{1}{r_2} - \dfrac{1}{n_1} - \dfrac{1}{n_2}}$	$RR = 0.12/0.25 = 0.48$ (48%); $\log(RR) = -0.734$; SE of $\log_e RR = \sqrt{\dfrac{1}{15} + \dfrac{1}{30} - \dfrac{1}{125} - \dfrac{1}{120}} = 0.289$; 95% CI for $\log_e RR$ is $-0.734 \pm 1.96 \times 0.289$, i.e. -1.301 to -0.167; 95% CI for RR is 0.272 to 0.846 or 27.2% to 84.6%
Relative risk reduction (RRR)	Not calculated	$RRR = 1 - RR = 1 - p_1/p_2 = 1 - 12/25 = 0.52$ (or 52%) 95% CI for RRR is obtained by subtracting CI for RR from 1 (or 100%), i.e. 0.154 to 0.728 or 15.4% to 72.8%

Odds ratio (OR)

$$OR = \frac{r_1(n_2 - r_2)}{r_2(n_1 - r_1)}$$

$$OR = \frac{15 \times 90}{30 \times 110} = 0.409; \log_e OR = -0.894$$

$$SE \text{ of } \log_e OR = \sqrt{\frac{1}{r_1} + \frac{1}{r_2} + \frac{1}{n_1 - r_1} + \frac{1}{n_2 - r_2}}$$

$$SE \text{ of } \log_e OR = \sqrt{\frac{1}{15} + \frac{1}{30} + \frac{1}{90} + \frac{1}{110}} = 0.347$$

95% CI for $\log_e OR$ is $-0.894 \pm 1.96 \times 0.347$, or -1.573 to -0.214; 95% CI for OR is 0.207 to 0.807

(c) Outcome is a measurement

Mean

If s is standard deviation (SD) of n observations, $SE = s/\sqrt{n}$

95% CI is mean $\pm t \times SE^f$

If mean = 17.2, s = 6.4, n = 38, then $SE = 6.4/\sqrt{38} = 1.038$ and 95% CI is $17.2 \pm 2.026 \times 1.038$ or 15.1 to 19.3

Difference between two means

If s_1 and s_2 are SDs of n_1 and n_2 observations, SE(diff) =

$$\sqrt{\frac{(n_1-1)s_1^2 + (n_2-1)s_2^2}{n_1 + n_2 - 2} \times \left(\frac{1}{n_1} + \frac{1}{n_2}\right)}$$

95% CI is mean difference $\pm t \times SE(\text{difference})^f$

If $mean_1 = 17.2$, $s_1 = 6.4$, $n_1 = 38$, $mean_2 = 15.9$, $s_2 = 5.6$, $n_2 = 45$, then mean difference = $d = 17.2 - 15.9$, = 1.3, t = 1.99^f

$$SE(\text{diff}) = \sqrt{\frac{37 \times 6.4^2 + 44 \times 5.6^2}{38 + 45 - 2} \times \left(\frac{1}{38} + \frac{1}{45}\right)} = 1.317$$

and 95% CIs is $1.3 \pm 1.99 \times 1.317$ or -1.32 to 3.92

Table A1-1 *(Cont'd)*

Clinical measure	Standard error (SE)	Typical calculation of SE and CI[a]
II. DIAGNOSTIC STUDIES		
(a) A single proportion		

In general, r diagnoses are observed among n patients, so the observed proportion is p = r/n. Using the notation of Chapter 3, the sensitivity is a/(a + c), the specificity is b/(b + d), the positive predictive value is a/(a + b), and the negative predictive value is d/(c + d).

The illustrative example is from Table 3.3. The sensitivity is 731/809 = 90% or 0.90, and the specificity is 1500/1770 = 85% or 0.85, p = 73/82 = 0.89 (or 89%).

| Sensitivity, specificity, predictive values | $SE = \sqrt{\dfrac{p \times (1-p)}{n}}$

 where p is proportion and n is number of patients | For the sensitivity, p = 731/809 = 0.90 (or 90%):

 $SE = \sqrt{\dfrac{0.90 \times 0.10}{809}} = 0.0105$ (or 1.05%)

 95% CI is 90% ± 1.96 × 1.05% or 87.9% to 92.1%[b] |

(b) Likelihood ratio

In general, the likelihood ratios for positive or negative test results are, respectively, obtained as either LR+ = sensitivity/(1 − specificity) and LR− = (1 − sensitivity)/specificity.

Likelihood ratio (LR)

$$LR+ = [a/(a + c)] / [b/(b + d)]$$
$$LR− = [c/(a + c)] / [d/(b + d)]$$

$$\text{SE of } \log_e LR+ = \sqrt{\frac{1}{a} + \frac{1}{b} - \frac{1}{(a+c)} - \frac{1}{(b+d)}}$$

$$\text{SE of } \log_e LR− = \sqrt{\frac{1}{c} + \frac{1}{d} - \frac{1}{(a+c)} - \frac{1}{(b+d)}}$$

$$LR+ = (731/809) / (270/1770) = 0.9/(1 − 0.85) = 6.0;$$
$$\log_e(LR+) = 1.792;$$

$$\text{SE of } \log_e LR+ = \sqrt{\frac{1}{731} + \frac{1}{270} - \frac{1}{809} - \frac{1}{1770}} = 0.0572;$$

95% CI for $\log_e LR+$ is 1.792 ± 1.96 × 0.0572,
i.e. 1.680 to 1.904; 95% CI for LR+ is 5.37 to 6.71
A similar approach is used to derive a CI for LR−

---

[a] In general a confidence interval is obtained by taking the estimate of interest and adding and subtracting a multiple of the SE. Except in the case of means or differences in means, the multiple is taken as a value from the standard normal distribution. For a 95% CI the multiplier is 1.96; for a 90% CI it is 1.645, and for a 99% CI it is 2.576. For proportions, this method is the traditional method referred to in footnote b. In some cases, such as for RR (and RRR) and OR, the CI is obtained for the logarithm of the quantity of interest and the values are antilogged (logs to base e are used in the table).

[b] The method illustrated is the traditional method. It works fine in most cases but is not recommended when sample sizes are small and/or proportions are near either 0% or 100% (in which case it is possible for the CI to include impossible values outside the range 0% to 100%). Newer methods are recommended both for general use and especially for the circumstances described. The methods are too complex to include here; they are described in reference 8 and incorporated into the software included with it.

[c] As used in this book, p_1 corresponds to the event rate in the experimental group (EER), and p_2 to the event rate in the control group (CER).

Table A1-1 (Cont'd)

d The above calculations assume that comparisons are between two independent groups. For CIs derived from paired data (e.g. from crossover trials or matched case–control studies), and also CIs for some other statistics, see reference 8.

e When the ARR is not significantly different from zero, one limit of the 95% CI is negative. Taking reciprocals gives a CI for the NNT with one negative value, which corresponds to a harmful effect. We can write the CI in terms of both the NNT and NNH. For example, a 95% CI for the ARR of −5% to 25% gives the 95% CI for the NNT of 10 as −20 to 4, or from NNH = 20 to NNT = 4. However, the values included in this interval are NNH from 20 to ∞ (infinity) and NNT from 4 to ∞. We can write this as NNH = 20 to ∞ to NNT = 4 (see references 8 and 9).

f The calculation of a CI for a mean or the difference between means uses the multiplier for a 95% CI is not 1.96 but a value from the t distribution with n − 1 or $n_1 + n_2 - 2$ degrees of freedom (df), respectively. The appropriate value of t is found from statistical tables or software. As df increases, t approaches 1.96. For df larger than 40, t is close to 2.

Figure A1.1 Relative risks of eclampsia for subgroups of women in a randomized trial of magnesium sulfate versus placebo for women with pre-eclampsia.[11] PMR, perinatal mortality rate.

Eclampsia Group	Relative risk (95% CI)	No. of events MgSO$_4$	Placebo
Severe pre-eclampsia	0.42 (0.23, 0.76)	15/1297	37/1345
Not severe pre-eclampsia	0.42 (0.26, 0.67)	25/3758	59/3710
Randomized before delivery	0.40 (0.27, 0.59)	36/4416	88/4359
... <34 weeks	0.54 (0.28, 1.06)	13/1206	24/1206
...>=34 weeks	0.35 (0.22, 0.57)	23/3210	64/3153
Randomized after delivery	0.54 (0.16, 1.80)	4/639	8/686
Anticonvulsant before trial	1.24 (0.49, 3.11)	10/439	8/435
No anticonvulsant before trial	0.34 (0.23, 0.51)	30/4590	88/4583
Imminent eclampsia	0.26 (0.12, 0.57)	8/810	31/829
No imminent eclampsia	0.49 (0.32, 0.75)	32/4245	65/4226
High PMR* country	0.34 (0.21, 0.56)	22/2814	64/2812
Middle PMR* country	0.54 (0.28, 1.03)	14/1463	26/1461
Low PMR* country	0.67 (0.19, 2.37)	4/778	6/782
ALL WOMEN	0.42 (0.29, 0.60)	40/5055	96/5055

*PMR: perinatal mortality rate.

273

eclampsia for subgroups of women in a placebo-controlled randomized trial of magnesium sulfate for women with pre-eclampsia.[11] The treatment effect is clearly consistent across subgroups except for a few subgroups with very few events.

In the same way, CIs are a key element of the standard "forest" plot used to display the results of each study in a systematic review.[12] Figure A1.2 shows the results of 11 RCTs of bovine rotavirus vaccine compared to placebo for preventing diarrhea.[13] The forest plot shows the estimated relative risk of diarrhea for each trial and the combined results from a meta-analysis (random effects). In each case a 95% CI is shown.

CLINICAL SIGNIFICANCE

I discussed above the error of taking lack of statistical significance as indicating that two treatments are equally effective. It is also important not to equate statistical significance with *clinical importance*. Clinical importance may be suggested when the result is statistically significant *and* estimated treatment effect exceeds some pre-specified amount (which may be the quantity used in the sample size calculation). A stricter criterion is that the whole CI should show benefit greater than the pre-specified minimum.

Studies can show results that may or may not be statistically significant, and which are or are not clinically important. In Figure A1.2, there are four trials for which the whole CI is below 1 and which thus have statistically significant results ($P < 0.05$): Christy, Clark (1988), Treanor and Vesikari (1985). Assuming that a clinically important difference would be a reduction of 20% in the risk of diarrhoea (RR = 0.8), all of these trials showed a clinically important estimated reduction in risk, but only for the study of Treanor is the whole 95% CI below this value. Two other trials—those of Mutz and Vesikari (1984)—showed clinically important results which were not statistically significant. Note that the three trials of Treanor, Vesikari (1984), and Vesikari (1985) had almost identical estimated treatment effects but differing widths of CI (reflecting sample size), and thus different strengths of

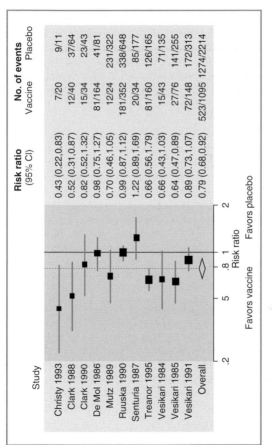

Figure A1.2 Forest plot showing results of 11 RCTs of bovine rotavirus vaccine compared to placebo for preventing diarrhea.[13] The plot for each trial shows the estimated relative risk of diarrhea with 95% CI; the size of the black square indicates the amount of information. Also shown is the pooled estimated treatment effect and 95% CI (shown as a diamond) from a random effects meta-analysis.

conclusions regarding both statistical significance and clinical importance when considered individually.

COMMENT

The most appropriate methods of statistical analysis and presentation must be largely a matter for personal judgment, although increasingly journals are requesting or requiring authors to use CIs when presenting their key findings. When the authors have not provided CIs, these can often be constructed using the results provided in their paper. While the focus in this appendix has been on RCTs, CIs are equally important for all study types.

The wide adoption of CIs in medical research papers has been of great benefit to a more correct understanding of the external evidence used in the practice of EBM. Nonetheless, it is common to see authors present CIs but ignore them when interpreting their results.[14] Readers should take note of CIs regardless of how authors interpret their study, and calculate them for themselves if authors fail to provide them.

REFERENCES

1 Gardner MJ, Altman DG. Confidence intervals rather than P values: estimation rather than hypothesis testing. BMJ 1986; 292: 746–50.

2 Rothman KJ, Yankauer A. Confidence intervals vs. significance tests: quantitative interpretation. Am J Public Health 1986; 76: 587–8.

3 Bulpitt CJ. Confidence intervals. Lancet 1986; i: 494–7.

4 Trollfors B, Taranger J, Lagergard T, et al. A placebo-controlled trial of a pertussis-toxoid vaccine. N Engl J Med 1995; 333: 1045–50.

5 Fallone CA, Mitchell A, Paterson WG. Determination of test performance of less costly methods of *Helicobacter pylori* detection. Clin Invest Med 1995; 18: 177–85.

6 Docherty JG, McGregor JR, Akyol AM, Murray GD, Galloway DJ. Comparison of manually constructed and stapled anastomoses in colorectal surgery. Ann Surg 1995; 221: 176–84.

7 Sung JJY, Chung SCS, Lai C-W, et al. Octreotide infusion or emergency sclerotherapy for variceal haemorrhage. Lancet 1993; 342: 637–41.

8 Altman DG, Machin D, Bryant TN, Gardner MJ, eds. Statistics with Confidence, 2nd edn. London: BMJ Books, 2000 (including CIA software).

9 Altman DG. Confidence intervals for the number needed to treat. BMJ 1998; 317: 1309–12.

10 Altman DG, Bland JM. Interaction revisited: the difference between two estimates. BMJ 2003; 326: 219.

11   The Magpie Trial Collaborative Group. Do women with pre-eclampsia, and their babies, benefit from magnesium sulphate? The Magpie Trial: a randomised placebo controlled trial. Lancet 2002; 359: 1877–90.

12   Lewis S, Clarke M. Forest plots: trying to see the wood and the trees. BMJ 2001; 322: 1479–80.

13   Soares-Weiser K, Goldberg E, Tamimi G, Pitan OC, Leibovici L. Rotavirus vaccine for preventing diarrhoea (Cochrane Review). The Cochrane Library, Issue 2. Chichester: Wiley, 2004.

14   Fidler F, Thomason N, Cumming G, Finch S, Leeman J. Editors can lead researchers to confidence intervals, but can't make them think: statistical reform lessons from medicine. Psychol Sci 2004; 15: 119–26.

Appendix 2: Glossary

TERMS YOU ARE LIKELY TO ENCOUNTER IN YOUR CLINICAL READING

Absolute risk reduction (ARR). See **treatment effects**.

Allocation concealment. Occurs when the person who is enrolling a participant into a clinical trial is unaware whether the next participant to be enrolled will be allocated to the intervention or control group.

Case–control study. A study which involves identifying patients who have the outcome of interest (cases) and control patients without the same outcome, and looking back to see if they had the exposure of interest.

Case series. A report on a series of patients with an outcome of interest. No control group is involved.

Clinical practice guideline. A systematically developed statement designed to assist clinician and patient decisions about appropriate health care for specific clinical circumstances.

Cohort study. Involves identification of two groups (cohorts) of patients, one that received the exposure of interest, and one that did not, and following these cohorts forward for the outcome of interest.

Confidence interval (CI). Quantifies the uncertainty in measurement. It is usually reported as 95% CI, which is the range of values within which we can be 95% sure that the true value for the whole population lies. For example, for an NNT of 10 with a 95% CI of 5 to 15, we would have 95% confidence that the true NNT value lies between 5 and 15.

Control event rate (CER). See **treatment effects**.

Cost–benefit analysis. Assesses whether the cost of an intervention is worth the benefit by measuring both in the same units; monetary units are usually used.

Cost-effectiveness analysis. Measures the net cost of providing an intervention as well as the outcomes obtained. Outcomes are reported in a single unit of measurement.

Cost-minimization analysis. If health effects are known to be equal, only costs are analyzed and the least costly alternative is chosen.

Cost–utility analysis. Converts health effects into personal preferences (or utilities) and describes how much it costs for some additional quality gain (e.g. cost per additional quality-adjusted life-year, or QALY).

Crossover study design. The administration of two or more experimental therapies one after the other in a specified or random order to the same group of patients.

Cross-sectional study. The observation of a defined population at a single point in time or time interval. Exposure and outcome are determined simultaneously.

Decision analysis (or clinical decision analysis). The application of explicit, quantitative methods that quantify prognoses, treatment effects, and patient values in order to analyze a decision under conditions of uncertainty.

Event rate. The proportion of patients in a group in whom the event is observed. Thus, if out of 100 patients, the event is observed in 27, the event rate is 0.27. Control event rate (CER) and experimental event rate (EER) are used to refer to this in control and experimental groups of patients, respectively. The patient expected event rate (PEER) refers to the rate of events we'd expect in a patient who received no treatment or conventional treatment. See **treatment effects**.

Evidence-based health care. Extends the application of the principles of evidence-based medicine (see below) to all professions associated with health care, including purchasing and management.

Evidence-based medicine (EBM). The conscientious, explicit, and judicious use of current best evidence in making decisions about the care of individual patients. The practice of evidence-based medicine requires the integration of individual clinical expertise with the best available external clinical evidence from systematic research and our patient's unique values and circumstances.

Experimental event rate (EER). See **treatment effects**.

Inception cohort. A group of patients who are assembled near the onset of the target disorder.

Incidence. The proportion of new cases of the target disorder in the population at risk during a specified time interval.

Intention-to-treat analysis. A method of analysis for randomized trials in which all patients randomly assigned to one of the treatments are analyzed together, regardless of whether or not they completed or received that treatment, in order to preserve randomization.

Likelihood ratio (LR). The likelihood that a given test result would be expected in a patient with the target disorder compared with the likelihood that the same result would be expected in a patient without the target disorder. See Table A2.2 for calculations.

Meta-analysis. A systematic review that uses quantitative methods to synthesize and summarize the results.

n-of-1 trials. In such trials, the patient undergoes pairs of treatment periods organized so that one period involves the use of the experimental treatment and the other involves the use of an alternate or placebo therapy. The patient and physician are blinded, if possible, and outcomes are monitored. Treatment periods are replicated until the clinician and patient are convinced that the treatments are definitely different or definitely not different.

Negative predictive value. Proportion of people with a negative test who are free of the target disorder. See also likelihood ratio.

Number needed to treat (NNT). The inverse of the absolute risk reduction and the number of patients that need to be treated to prevent one bad outcome. See **treatment effects**.

Odds. A ratio of the number of people incurring an event to the number of people who don't have an event.

Odds ratio (OR). The ratio of the odds of having the target disorder in the experimental group relative to the odds in favor of having the target disorder in the control group (in cohort studies or systematic reviews), or the odds in favor of being exposed in participants with the target disorder divided by the odds in favor of being exposed in control participants (without the target disorder). See Table A2.4 for calculations.

Overview. See systematic review.

Patient expected event rate (PEER). See treatment effects.

Positive predictive value. Proportion of people with a positive test who have the target disorder. See also **likelihood ratio**.

Post-test odds. The odds that the patient has the target disorder after the test is carried out [(pre-test odds) × (likelihood ratio)].

Post-test probability. The proportion of patients with that particular test result who have the target disorder [(post-test odds)/(1 + post-test odds)].

Pre-test odds. The odds that the patient has the target disorder before the test is carried out [(pre-test probability)/(1 − pre-test probability)].

Pre-test probability/prevalence. The proportion of people with the target disorder in the population at risk at a specific time (point prevalence) or time interval (period prevalence). See also **likelihood ratio**.

Randomization (or random allocation). Method analogous to tossing a coin to assign patients to treatment groups (the experimental treatment is assigned if the coin lands "heads"; a conventional, "control" or "placebo" treatment is given if the coin lands "tails").

Randomized controlled clinical trial (RCT). Participants are randomly allocated into an experimental group or a control group and followed over time for the variables/outcomes of interest.

Relative risk reduction (RRR). See treatment effects.

Risk ratio (RR). The ratio of the risk in the treated group (EER) to the risk in the control group (CER); used in randomized trials and cohort studies. RR = ERR/CER. Also called relative risk.

Sensitivity. Proportion of people with the target disorder who have a positive test result. It is used to assist in assessing and selecting a diagnostic test/sign/symptom. See also **likelihood ratio**.

SnNout. When a sign/test/symptom has a high sensitivity (**Sn**), a negative result (**N**) can help rule out (**out**) the diagnosis. For example, the sensitivity of a history of ankle swelling for diagnosing ascites is 93%; therefore, if a person does not have a history of ankle swelling, it is highly unlikely that the person has ascites.

Specificity. Proportion of people without the target disorder who have a negative test result. It is used to assist in assessing and selecting a diagnostic test/sign/symptom. See also **likelihood ratio**.

SpPin. When a sign/test/symptom has a high specificity (**Sp**), a positive result (**P**) can help to rule in (**in**) the diagnosis. For example, the specificity of a fluid wave for diagnosing ascites is 92%; therefore, if a person does have a fluid wave, he/she may have ascites.

Systematic review. A summary of the medical literature that uses explicit methods to perform a comprehensive literature search and critical appraisal of individual studies, and that uses appropriate statistical techniques to combine these valid studies.

Treatment effects. The evidence-based journals (*Evidence Based Medicine* and *ACP Journal Club*) have achieved consensus on some of the terms they use to describe both the good and the bad effects of therapy. We will bring them to life with a synthesis of three randomized trials in diabetes which individually showed that several years of intensive insulin therapy reduced the proportion of patients with worsening retinopathy to 13% from 38%, raised the proportion of patients with satisfactory hemoglobin A_{1c} levels to 60% from about 30%, and increased the proportion of patients with at least one episode of symptomatic hypoglycemia to 57%

from 23%. Note that, in each case, the first number constitutes the "experimental event rate" (EER), and the second number the "control event rate" (CER). We will use the following terms and calculations to describe these effects of treatment.

When the experimental treatment reduces the probability of a bad outcome (worsening diabetic retinopathy)

RRR (relative risk reduction). The proportional reduction in rates of bad outcomes between experimental and control participants in a trial, calculated as $|\text{EER} - \text{CER}|/\text{CER}$, and accompanied by a 95% confidence interval (CI). In the case of worsening diabetic retinopathy, $|\text{EER} - \text{CER}|/\text{CER}$ $= |13\% - 38\%|/38\% = 66\%$.

ARR (absolute risk reduction). The absolute arithmetic difference in rates of bad outcomes between experimental and control participants in a trial, calculated as $|\text{EER} - \text{CER}|$, and accompanied by a 95% CI. In this case, $|\text{EER} - \text{CER}| = |13\% - 38\%| = 25\%$. (This is sometimes called the risk difference.)

NNT (number needed to treat). The number of patients who need to be treated to achieve one additional favorable outcome, calculated as 1/ARR and accompanied by a 95% CI. In this case, $1/\text{ARR} = 1/25\% = 4$.

When the experimental treatment increases the probability of a good outcome (satisfactory hemoglobin A_{1c} levels)

RBI (relative benefit increase). The proportional increase in rates of good outcomes between experimental and control patients in a trial, calculated as $|\text{EER} - \text{CER}|/\text{CER}$, and accompanied by a 95% confidence interval (CI). In the case of satisfactory hemoglobin A_{1c} levels, $|\text{EER} - \text{CER}|/\text{CER} = |60\% - 30\%|/30\% = 100\%$.

ABI (absolute benefit increase). The absolute arithmetic difference in rates of good outcomes between experimental and control patients in a trial, calculated as $|\text{EER} - \text{CER}|$, and accompanied by a 95% CI. In the case of satisfactory hemoglobin A_{1c} levels, $|\text{EER} - \text{CER}| = |60\% - 30\%| = 30\%$

NNT (number needed to treat). The number of patients who need to be treated to achieve one additional good outcome, calculated as 1/ARR and accompanied by a 95% CI. In this case, 1/ARR = 1/30% = 3.

When the experimental treatment increases the probability of a bad outcome (episodes of hypoglycemia)

RRI (relative risk increase). The proportional increase in rates of bad outcomes between experimental and control patients in a trial, calculated as $|EER - CER|/CER$, and accompanied by a 95% confidence interval (CI). In the case of hypoglycemic episodes, $|EER - CER|/CER = |57\% - 23\%|/23\% = 148\%$. (RRI is also used in assessing the impact of "risk factors" for disease.)

ARI (absolute risk increase). The absolute arithmetic difference in rates of bad outcomes between experimental and control patients in a trial, calculated as $|EER - CER|$, and accompanied by a 95% CI. In the case of hypoglycemic episodes, $|EER - CER| = |57\% - 23\%| = 34\%$. (ARI is also used in assessing the impact of "risk factors" for disease.)

NNH (number needed to harm). The number of patients who, if they received the experimental treatment, would result in one additional patient being harmed, compared with patients who received the control treatment; calculated as 1/ARR and accompanied by a 95% CI. In this case, 1/ARR = 1/34% = 3.

Table A2.1

Occurrence of diabetic retinopathy at 5 years among insulin-dependent diabetics		Relative risk reduction	Absolute risk reduction	NNT
Usual insulin regimen (CER)	Intensive insulin regimen (EER)	$\dfrac{(|EER - CER|)}{CER}$	$|EER - CER|$	1/ARR
38%	13%	$|13\% - 38\%|/38\%$ $= 68\%$	$|13\% - 38\%|$ $= 25\%$	1/25% $= 4$ patients

How to calculate LRs

Table A2.2			
Diagnostic test result	Target disorder		
+	a	b	a + b
−	c	d	c + d
	a + c	b + d	a + b + c + d

We can assume that there are four possible groups of patients, as indicated (a to d) in the table. From these we can determine the "sensitivity" and "specificity" as follows:

$$\text{Sensitivity} = a/(a + c)$$
$$\text{Specificity} = d/(b + d)$$

We can now use these to calculate the likelihood ratio for a positive test result (LR+):

$$\text{LR+} = \text{sensitivity}/(1 - \text{specificity})$$
$$= [a/(a + c)]/[b/(b + d)]$$

Similarly, we can calculate the likelihood ratio for a negative test result (LR−):

$$\text{LR−} = (1 - \text{sensitivity})/\text{specificity}$$
$$= [c/(a + c)]/[d/(b + d)]$$

Positive predictive value = $a/(a + b)$
Negative predictive value = $d/(c + d)$
Pre-test probability = $(a + c)/(a + b + c + d)$

SAMPLE CALCULATION

Suppose you have a patient with anemia and a serum ferritin of 60 mmol/L. You come across a systematic review[*] of serum ferritin as a diagnostic test for iron deficiency anemia, with the results summarized in the following table.

---

[*] J Gen Intern Med 1992; 7: 145–53.

Table A2.3

Diagnostic test result (serum ferritin)	Target disorder (iron deficiency anemia)		Totals
	Present	Absent	
+ (<65 mmol/L)	731	270	1001
	a	b	a + b
− (≥65 mmol/L)	78	1500	1578
	c	d	c + d
	809	1770	2579
	a + c	b + d	a + b + c + d

These results indicate that 90% of the patients with iron deficiency anemia have a positive test result (serum ferritin <65 mmol/L). This is known as the "sensitivity" and is calculated as:

$$\text{Sensitivity} = a/(a + c) = 731/809 = 90\%$$

The results also show that 85% of patients who do not have iron deficiency anemia have a negative test result. This is referred to as the "specificity", calculated as:

$$\text{Specificity} = d/(b + d) = 1500/1770 = 85\%$$

From the sensitivity and specificity, the positive (LR+) and negative (LR−) likelihood ratios can be determined:

$$\text{LR+} = \text{sensitivity}/(1 - \text{specificity}) = 90\%/15\% = 6$$
$$\text{LR−} = (1 - \text{sensitivity})/\text{specificity} = 10\%/85\% = 0.12$$

Thus, from your calculation of LR+, you determine that your patient's positive test result would be about six times more likely to be seen in someone with iron deficiency anemia than in someone without the disorder.

CALCULATION OF ODDS RATIO/RELATIVE RISK

The table below can be used to calculate the odds ratio/relative risk for the use of trimethoprim–sulfamethoxazole prophylaxis in cirrhosis:

Table A2.4			
	Adverse event occurs (infectious complication)	Adverse event doesn't occur (no infectious complication)	Totals
Exposed to treatment (experimental)	1 a	29 b	30 a + b
Not exposed to treatment (control)	9 c	21 d	30 c+d
Totals	10 a + c	50 b + d	60 a + b + c + d

$CER = c/(c + d) = 0.30$
$EER = a/(a + b) = 0.033$
Control event odds $= c/d = 0.43$
Experimental event odds $= a/b = 0.034$
Relative risk $= EER/CER = 0.11$
Relative odds $=$ odds ratio $= (a/b)/(c/d) = ad/bc = 0.08$

Index

Page numbers in **bold** type refer to figures; those in *italic* to tables.

Card 8A HARM/ETIOLOGY

Is this evidence about harm valid?

1. Were there clearly defined groups of patients, similar in all important ways other than exposure to the treatment or other cause?
2. Were treatments/exposures and clinical outcomes measured in the same ways in both groups? (Was the assessment of outcomes either objective or blinded to exposure?)
3. Was the follow-up of the study patients sufficiently long (for the outcome to occur) and complete?
4. Do the results of the harm study fulfill some of the diagnostic tests for causation?
   - Is it clear that the exposure preceded the onset of the outcome?
   - Is there a dose–response gradient?
   - Is there any positive evidence from a "dechallenge–rechallenge" study?
   - Is the association consistent from study to study?
   - Does the association make biological sense?

Is this valid evidence about harm important?

	Adverse outcome		Totals
	Present (case)	Absent (controls)	
Exposed to treatment (RCT or cohort)	a	b	a + b
Not exposed to treatment (RCT or cohort)	c	d	c + d
Totals	a + c	b + d	a + b + c + d

- In a randomized trial or cohort study: relative risk (RR) = $[a/(a + b)]/[c/(c + d)]$.
- In a case-control study: relative odds = ad/bc.

1. What is the magnitude of the association between the exposure and outcome?
2. What is the precision of the estimate of the association between the exposure and the outcome?

To convert odds ratio (or relative odds) to an NNH:
NNH = $1 + [PEER \times (OR - 1)]/(1 - PEER) \times (PEER) \times (OR - 1)$

From Straus, Richardson, Glasziou, Haynes: Evidence-Based Medicine; How to Practice and Teach EBM. Elsevier, Edinburgh, 2005

Card 8B HARM/ETIOLOGY

NNHs derived from typical PEERs and ORs[a]

		For odds ratios LESS than 1						
		0.9	0.8	0.7	0.6	0.5	0.4	0.3
Patient	0.05	209	104	69	52	41	34	29
expected	0.10	110	54	36	27	21	18	15
event	0.20	61	30	20	14	11	10	8
rate	0.30	46	22	14	10	8	7	5
(PEER)	0.40	40	19	12	9	7	6	4
	0.50[a]	38	18	11	8	6	5	4
	0.70	44	20	13	9	6	5	4
	0.90	101	46	27	18	12	9	4

		For odds ratios GREATER than 1						
		1.1	1.25	1.5	1.75	2	2.25	2.5
Patient	0.05	212	86	44	30	23	18	16
expected	0.10	113	46	24	16	13	10	9
event	0.20	64	27	14	10	8	7	6
rate	0.30	50	21	11	8	7	6	5
(PEER)	0.40	44	19	10	8	6	5	5
	0.50	42	18	10	8	6	6	5
	0.70	51	23	13	10	9	8	7
	0.90	121	55	33	25	22	19	18

[a]Adapted from John Geddes, 1999

Can we apply the valid, important results of this harm study to our patient?

1. Is our patient so different from those included in the study that its results cannot apply?
2. What is our patient's risk of benefit and harm from the agent?
3. What are our patient's preferences, concerns and expectations from this treatment?
4. What alternative treatments are available?

From Straus, Richardson, Glasziou, Haynes: *Evidence-Based Medicine: How to Practice and Teach EBM*. Elsevier, Edinburgh, 2005

Card 1A **DIAGNOSIS**

Is this evidence about diagnosis valid?

1. Was there an independent, blind comparison with a reference ("gold") standard of diagnosis?
2. Was the diagnostic test evaluated in an appropriate spectrum of patients (like those in whom it would be used in practice)?
3. Was the reference standard applied regardless of the diagnostic test result?
4. Was the cluster of tests validated in a second, independent group of patients?

Is this valid evidence about diagnosis important?

		Target disorder (iron deficiency anemia)		Totals
		Present	Absent	
Diagnostic test result (serum ferritin)	Positive (<65 mmol/L)	731 a	270 b	1001 a + b
	Negative (≥65 mmol/L)	c 78	d 1500	c + d 1578
	Totals	a + c 809	b + d 1770	a + b + c + d 2579

Sensitivity = $a/(a + c)$ = 731/809 = 90%.
Specificity = $d/(b + d)$ = 1500/1770 = 85%.

Likelihood ratio for a positive test result = LR+ = sensitivity/$(1 - \text{specificity})$ = 90%/15% = 6.
Likelihood ratio for a negative test result = LR− = $(1 - \text{sensitivity})/\text{specificity}$ = 10%/85% = 0.12.
Positive predictive value = $a/(a + b)$ = 731/1001 = 73%.
Negative predictive value = $d/(c + d)$ = 1500/1578 = 95%.
Pre-test probability (prevalence) = $(a + c)/(a + b + c + d)$ = 809/2579 = 31%.
Pre-test odds = prevalence/$(1 - \text{prevalence})$ = 31%/69% = 0.45.
Post-test odds = pre-test odds × likelihood ratio.
Post-test probability = post-test odds/(post-test odds + 1).

Can we apply this valid, important evidence about a diagnostic test in caring for our patient?

1. Is the diagnostic test available, affordable, accurate, and precise in our setting?
2. Can we generate a clinically sensible estimate of our patient's pre-test probability?
   - From personal experience, prevalence statistics, practice databases, or primary studies
   - Are the study patients similar to our own?
   - Is it unlikely that the disease possibilities or probabilities have changed since this evidence was gathered?
3. Will the resulting post-test probabilities affect our management and help our patient?
   - Could it move us across a test–treatment threshold?
   - Would our patient be a willing partner in carrying it out?
   - Would the consequences of the test help our patient reach his or her goals in all this?

From Straus, Richardson, Glasziou, Haynes: Evidence-Based Medicine; How to Practice and Teach EBM. Elsevier, Edinburgh, 20

Card 1B DIAGNOSIS

Diagnostic usefulness of five levels of a test result

Diagnostic test result	Serum ferritin (mmol/L)	Target disorder (iron deficiency) present		Target disorder absent		Likelihood ratio	Diagnostic impact
		Number	%	Number	%		
Very positive	<15	474	59% (474/809)	20	1.1% (20/1770)	52	Rule in "SpPin"
Moderately positive	15–34	175	22% (175/809)	79	4.5% (79/1770)	4.8	Intermediate high
Neutral	35–64	82	10% (82/809)	171	10% (171/1770)	1	Intermediate
Moderately negative	65–94	30	3.7% (30/809)	168	9.5% (168/1770)	0.39	Intermediate low
Extremely negative	≥95	48	5.9% (48/809)	1332	75% (1332/1770)	0.08	Rule out "SnNout"
Totals		809	100% (809/809)	1770	100% (1770/1770)		

From Straus, Richardson, Glasziou, Haynes: Evidence-Based Medicine; How to Practice and Teach EBM. Elsevier, Edinburgh, 2005

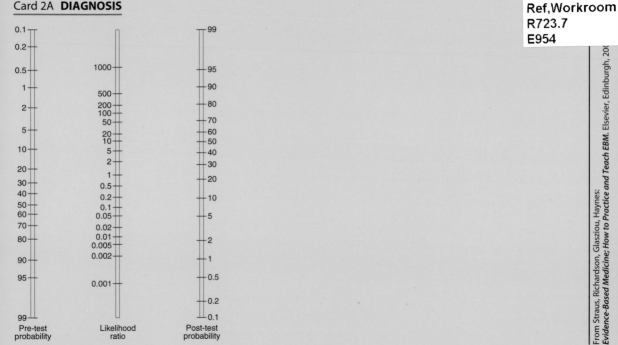

A likelihood ratio nomogram.

From Straus, Richardson, Glasziou, Haynes: *Evidence-Based Medicine; How to Practice and Teach EBM*. Elsevier, Edinburgh, 200

PRE-TEST PROBABILITY

Is this evidence about pre-test probability valid?

1. Did the study patients represent the full spectrum of those who present with this clinical problem?
2. Were the criteria for each final diagnosis explicit and credible?
3. Was the diagnostic work-up comprehensive and consistently applied?
4. For initially undiagnosed patients, was follow-up sufficiently long and complete?

Is this valid evidence about pre-test probability important?

1. What were the diagnoses and their probabilities?
2. How precise were these estimates of disease probability?

SCREENING AND CASE-FINDING

Guides for deciding whether a screening or case-finding maneuver does more good than harm

1. Is there RCT evidence that early diagnosis really leads to improved survival, or quality of life, or both?
2. Are the early-diagnosed patients willing partners in the treatment strategy?
3. How do benefits and harms compare in different people and with different screening strategies?
4. Do the frequency and severity of the target disorder warrant the degree of effort and expenditure?

From Straus, Richardson, Glasziou, Haynes: *Evidence-Based Medicine; How to Practice and Teach EBM.* Elsevier, Edinburgh, 2005

Card 3A THERAPY (single trials)

Is this evidence about therapy valid?

1. Was the assignment of patients to treatment randomized?
2. Was the randomization concealed?
3. Were the groups similar at the start of the trial?
4. Was follow-up of patients sufficiently long and complete?
5. Were all patients analyzed in the groups to which they were randomized?

Some finer points:

6. Were patients, clinicians and study personnel kept blind to treatment?
7. Were groups treated equally, apart from the experimental therapy?

Is this valid evidence about therapy important?

	Event rate = stroke (mean follow-up 5 years)		Relative risk reduction (RRR)	Absolute risk reduction (ARR)	Number needed to treat (NNT)
	Control rate (CER)	Experimental event rate (EER)	|CER − EER|/CER	|CER − EER|	1/ARR
MRC trial	5.7%	4.3%	|5.7% − 4.3%|/5.7% = 25%	|5.7% − 4.3%| = 0.014 or 1.4%	1/1.4% = 72
Hypothetical, trivial case	0.000057%	0.000043%	|0.000057% − 0.000043%|/0.000057% = 25%	|0.000057% − 0.000043%| = 0.000014%	1/0.000014% = 7142857

1. What is the magnitude of the treatment effect?
2. How precise is the estimate of the treatment effect?

Can we apply this valid, important evidence about therapy in caring for our patient?

1. Is our patient so different from those in the study that its results cannot apply?
2. Is the treatment feasible in our setting?
3. What are our patient's potential benefits and harms from the therapy?
4. What are our patient's values and expectations for both the outcome we are trying to prevent and the treatment we are offering?

From Straus, Richardson, Glasziou, Haynes: *Evidence-Based Medicine; How to Practice and Teach EBM.* Elsevier, Edinburgh, 2

Card 3B **THERAPY**

Guides for whether to believe apparent qualitative differences in the efficacy of therapy in some subgroups of patients

A qualitative difference in treatment efficacy among subgroups is likely only when ALL the following questions can be answered "yes":
1. Does it really make biological and clinical sense?
2. Is the qualitative difference both clinically (beneficial for some but useless or harmful for others) and statistically significant?
3. Was it hypothesized before the study began (rather than the product of dredging the data)?
4. Was it one of just a few subgroup analyses carried out in the study?
5. Has the result been confirmed in other independent studies?

The likelihood of help vs. harm (LHH)

In applying a systematic review or RCT to an individual patient, we need to consider:
- Our patient's risk, relative to patients in the trial, of the event we hope to prevent with the treatment: f_t.
- Our patient's risk, relative to patients in the trial, of the side-effect we might cause from the treatment: f_h.
- Our patient's perception of the severity of the event we're trying to prevent relative to the side-effect we might cause: s.

The likelihood of help vs. harm is $(1/NNT) \times f_t \times s$ vs. $(1/NNH) \times f_h$

For example, suppose we're applying a trial with an NNT of 9 and an NNH of 12 and we think our patient is at just half the risk of the event but at twice the risk of the side-effect, then the "raw" LHH before we adjust it for our patient's perception of relative severity is $1/9 \times 0.5$ vs. $1/12 \times 2 = 1/18$ vs. 1/6, or three times as likely to harm vs. help the patient. However, if our patient regards the severity of the event that the treatment might prevent to be six times worse than the side-effect it might cause, then the final LHH $= 1/18 \times 6$ vs. 1/6, or two times as likely to help vs. harm.

From Straus, Richardson, Glasziou, Haynes: *Evidence-Based Medicine; How to Practice and Teach EBM.* Elsevier, Edinburgh, 2005

Card 4A THERAPY: SYSTEMATIC REVIEWS

Are the results of this systematic review of therapy valid?
1. Is this a systematic review of randomized trials?
2. Does it describe a comprehensive and detailed search for relevant trials?
3. Were the individual studies assessed for validity?

A less-frequent point:
4. Were individual patient data (or aggregate data) used in the analysis?

Are the valid results of this systematic review of therapy important?
1. Are the results consistent across studies?
2. What is the magnitude of the treatment effect?
3. How precise is the treatment effect?

Translating odds ratios (ORs) to NNTs

1. When the odds ratio (OR) < 1. The numbers in the body of the table are the NNTs for the corresponding odds ratios at that particular patient's expected event rate (PEER). This table applies when a bad outcome is prevented by therapy.

		OR < 1				
		0.9	0.8	0.7	0.6	0.5
Patient's	0.05	209[a]	104	69	52	41[b]
expected	0.10	110	54	36	27	21
event	0.20	61	30	20	14	11
rate	0.30	46	22	14	10	8
(PEER)	0.40	40	19	12	9	7
	0.50	38	18	11	9	6
	0.70	44	20	13	9	6
	0.90	101[c]	46	27	18	12[d]

[a]The relative risk reduction (RRR) here is 10%.
[b]The RRR here is 49%.
[c]The RRR here is 1%.
[d]The RRR here is 9%.

2. When the odds ratio (OR) > 1. The numbers in the body of the table are the NNTs are for the corresponding odds ratios at that particular patient's expected event rate (PEER). This table applies both when a good outcome is increased by therapy and when a side-effect is caused by therapy.

		OR > 1				
		1.1	1.2	1.3	1.4	1.5
Patient's	0.05	212	106	71	54	43
expected	0.10	112	57	38	29	23
event	0.20	64	33	22	17	14
rate	0.30	49	25	17	13	11
(PEER)	0.40	43	23	16	12	10
	0.50	42	22	15	12	10
	0.70	51	27	19	15	13
	0.90	121	66	47	38	32

From Straus, Richardson, Glasziou, Haynes: *Evidence-Based Medicine; How to Practice and Teach EBM.* Elsevier, Edinburgh, 20

Card 4B SYSTEMATIC REVIEWS

Formulae to convert odds ratios (ORs) and relative risks (RRs) to NNTs

For RR <1:
$$NNT = 1/(1 - RR) \times PEER$$
For RR >1:
$$NNT = 1/(RR - 1) \times PEER$$

For OR <1:
$$NNT = 1 - [PEER \times (1 - OR)]/(1 - PEER) \times (PEER) \times (1 - OR)$$
For OR >1:
$$NNT = 1 + [PEER \times (OR - 1)]/(1 - PEER) \times (PEER) \times (OR - 1)$$

Can we apply this valid, important evidence about therapy in caring for our patient?

1. Is our patient so different from those in the study that its results cannot apply?
2. Is the treatment feasible in our setting?
3. What are our patient's potential benefits and harms from the therapy?
4. What are our patient's values and expectations for both the outcome we are trying to prevent and the adverse effects we may cause?

From Straus, Richardson, Glasziou, Haynes: *Evidence-Based Medicine; How to Practice and Teach EBM.* Elsevier, Edinburgh, 2005

Card 5A CLINICAL DECISION ANALYSIS

Is this evidence from a CDA valid?

1. Were all important therapeutic alternatives (including no treatment) and outcomes included?
2. Are the probabilities of the outcomes valid and credible?
3. Are the utilities of the outcomes valid and credible?

Is this valid evidence from a CDA important?

1. Did one course of action lead to clinically important gains?
2. Was the same course of action preferred despite clinically sensible changes in probabilities and utilities?

Can we apply these valid, important results of the CDA to our patient?

1. Do the probabilities in this CDA apply to our patient?
2. Can our patient state his/her utilities in a stable, usable form?

From Straus, Richardson, Glasziou, Haynes: *Evidence-Based Medicine; How to Practice and Teach EBM.* Elsevier, Edinburgh, 2005

Card 5B ECONOMIC ANALYSIS

Is this evidence from an economic analysis valid?

1. Are all well-defined courses of action compared?
2. Does it provide a specified view from which the costs and consequences are being viewed?
3. Does it cite comprehensive evidence on the efficacy of alternatives?
4. Does it identify all the costs and consequences we think it should and select credible and accurate measures of them?
5. Was the type of analysis appropriate for the question posed?

Is this valid evidence from an economic analysis important?

1. Are the resulting costs or cost/unit of health gained clinically significant?
2. Did the results of this economic analysis change with sensible changes to costs and effectiveness?

Can we apply the valid, important results of this economic analysis to our patient?

1. Do the costs in the economic analysis apply in our setting?
2. Are the treatments likely to be effective in our setting?

From Straus, Richardson, Glasziou, Haynes: *Evidence-Based Medicine; How to Practice and Teach EBM.* Elsevier, Edinburgh, 2005

Card 6A GUIDELINES

Are the recommendations in this guideline valid?

1. Did its developers carry out a comprehensive, reproducible literature review within the past 12 months?
2. Is each of its recommendations both tagged by the level of evidence upon which it is based and linked to a specific citation?

The killer Bs

1. Is the **B**urden of illness (frequency in our community, or our patient's pre-test probability or expected event rate [PEER]) too low to warrant implementation?
2. Are the **B**eliefs of individual patients or communities about the value of the interventions or their consequences incompatible with the guideline?
3. Would the opportunity cost of implementing this guideline constitute a bad **B**argain in the use of our energy or our community's resources?
4. Are the **B**arriers (geographic, organizational, traditional, authoritarian, legal, or behavioral) so high that it is not worth trying to overcome them?

From Straus, Richardson, Glasziou, Haynes:
Evidence-Based Medicine; How to Practice and Teach EBM. Elsevier, Edinburgh, 2005

Card 6B QUALITATIVE RESEARCH

IS THE EVIDENCE FROM THIS QUALITATIVE STUDY VALID, IMPORTANT AND APPLICABLE?

Is the evidence from this qualitative study valid?

1. Was the selection of participants explicit and appropriate?
2. Were the methods for data collection and analysis explicit and appropriate?

Is the valid evidence from this qualitative study important?

1. Are the results impressive?

Is the valid and important evidence from this qualitative study applicable to my patient?

1. Do these same phenomena apply to my patient?

From Straus, Richardson, Glasziou, Haynes: *Evidence-Based Medicine; How to Practice and Teach EBM.* Elsevier, Edinburgh, 2005

Card 7A PROGNOSIS

Is this evidence about prognosis valid?

1. Was a defined, representative sample of patients assembled at a common point in the course of their disease?
2. Was follow-up of study patients sufficiently long and complete?
3. Were objective outcome criteria applied in a "blind" fashion?

If subgroups with different prognoses are identified:
- Was there adjustment for important prognostic factors?
- Was there validation in an independent group of "test-set" patients?

Is this valid evidence about prognosis important?

1. How likely are the outcomes over time?
2. How precise are the prognostic estimates?

Can we apply this valid, important evidence about prognosis to our patient?

1. Is our patient so different from those in the study that its results cannot apply?
2. Will this evidence make a clinically important impact on our conclusions about what to offer or tell our patient?

From Straus, Richardson, Glasziou, Haynes: *Evidence-Based Medicine; How to Practice and Teach EBM*. Elsevier, Edinburgh, 2005

Card 7B **USEFUL URLs**

- **The book:** www.cebm.utoronto.ca
- **Netting the evidence** (list of EBM resources, including websites, etc.): http://www.shef.ac.uk/~scharr/ir/netting/
- **PubMed Clinical Queries:** http://www.ncbi.nlm.nih.gov/entrez/query/static/clinical.html
- **The Cochrane Library:** www.cochrane.org
- **ACP Journal Club:** www.acpjc.org
- **EBM Journal:** http://ebm.bmjjournals.com/
- **NHS R&D Centre for EBM in Oxford** (including a schedule of EBM workshops): www.cebm.net
- **EPIQ:** http://www.epiq.co.nz
- **Ovid:** http://www.ovid.com
- **For health services research topics** (the appropriateness, process, and outcomes of health services, and clinical practice guidelines): http://www.nlm.nih.gov/nichsr/hedges/search.html

From Straus, Richardson, Glasziou, Haynes; *Evidence-Based Medicine; How to Practice and Teach EBM.* Elsevier, Edinburgh, 2005